The
Potent Power
of
Menopause

BOOKS ALSO BY DAWN BATES

Becoming Annie – The Biography of a Curious Woman
by Dawn Bates (2020)

Friday Bridge – Becoming a Muslim, Becoming Everyone's Business
(2nd Edition, 2017)

Walaahi – A firsthand account of living through the Egyptian Uprising
and why I walked away from Islaam (2017)

Crossing The Line – A Journey of Purpose and Self-Belief (2017)

The Sacral Series by Dawn Bates:

Moana – One Woman's Journey Back to Self (2020)

Leila – A Life Renewed One Canvas at a Time (2020)

Pandora – Melting the Ice One Dive at a Time (2021)

Alpha – Saving Humanity One Vagina at a Time (2021)

ALSO PUBLISHED BY DAWN PUBLISHING:

Becoming the Champion – V1 Awareness
by Korey Carpenter (2020)

Break Down to Wake Up – Journey Beyond the Now
by Jocelyn Bellows (2020)

Unlocked – Discover Your Hidden Keys
by Carmelle Crinnion (2020)

Standing in Strength – Inspirational Stories of Power Unleashed (2021)

The Recipe – A US Marine's Mindset for Success (2021)

The Democ-chu Series by Nath Brye:

Slave Boy (2020)

Blood Child (2021)

A CULTURALLY DIVERSE
PERSPECTIVE OF
FEMININE **TRANSFORMATION**

The
Potent Power
of
Menopause

Curated by
DAWN BATES
&
CLARISSA KRISTJANSSON

© 2022 Dawn Bates & Clarissa Kristjansson

Published by Dawn Publishing
www.dawnbates.com
The moral right of the authors has been asserted.

For quantity sales or media enquiries, please contact the publisher at the website address above.

Cataloguing-in-Publication entry is available from the British Library.

ISBN: 978-1-913973-18-6 (paperback)
        978-1-913973-19-3 (ebook)

Book cover design – Alexander Von Ness

To discover more about Dawn Bates, the founder of Dawn Publishing, and the latest book releases, competitions and offers make sure you sign up for her regular weekly-ish emails using https://dawnbates.com/dive-in

Are you a writer? Do you want to get published? Then make sure you visit the home of Dawn Publishing at https://dawnbates.com/writers and see how Dawn can help you on your journey to becoming published!

We dedicate this book to the women of the world, past, present and future. May you love your body, own your sovereignty and harness your feminine power for the greatness of self, and humanity.

As a thank you for purchasing this book, Dawn is inviting you to take part in her powerful transformation programme The 21 Day Phoenix UpRising Lifestyle Reboot. It is packed full of ideas on how to create your new vision for the future, and will take you less than one hour a day. It is designed for YOU! The woman who wants to create powerful change her life – regardless of what stage you are at and where you wish to BE. When you enter the following coupon code: menopause – you will receive a special discounted rate. So click on this link and get your gift!
https://www.learndesk.us/class/6485771030626304/phoenix-uprising-21-day-lifestyle-reboot

Clarissa is also inviting you to take part in her powerful course: 'My Mindful Menopause' which will equip you with mindfulness tools and techniques that help you to manage your menopause symptoms. It will support you to feel calmer, more in control and empowered to go through menopause.
https://clarissa-s-school-f0dd.thinkific.com/courses/mindfulmenopause

CONTENTS

Gratitude

Any project which spans the world's time zones and continents takes patience, determination and resilience. When that project includes diving deep into the core of who we are, combined with opening up about a personal journey and sharing it with the world, it takes courage and the willingness to be open and vulnerable.

We send gratitude to all of our fellow co-authors on this project who have entrusted us to bring their stories to the world.

We would also like to send gratitude to the team behind the scenes who have put so much into bringing this book to the market.

Gratitude is also sent to all who have shared their journeys publicly and privately so we can break through the shame and stigma of menopause and link arms in sisterhood.

With love,

Dawn and Clarissa

Introduction

Back in 2018 during a conversation with a friend back in the UK, she mentioned the perimenopause, starting off a chain of thoughts within my mind.

These thoughts led to the curiosity of wanting to understand the menopause with even more depth - just to make sure the high achiever within me knew what to expect so I could plan effectively and succeed.

Succeed at what I wasn't sure, but succeed at this menopause malarkey I would, because failure is not an option in my world.

As I started this journey of discovery, I became bored, depressed and uninterested because the books were clinical, boring and didn't offer much hope or humour.

And I for one love to laugh, so much so my motto in life is: 'Live to laugh and laugh to live'.

Arriving on land after three months at sea crossing the Atlantic Ocean, I had been booked to appear on a podcast hosted by none other than Clarissa Kristjansson - Menopause Guru Extraordinaire.

My journaling was yet again proving to provide the results in life I wanted!

I instantly felt a great connection with Clarissa and knew she was the woman I wanted to learn from. And giggle with.

The idea for this book had already formed in my mind, because I was sure that I was not the only one who wanted to laugh whilst learning about the incredible transformation our bodies go through on our journey to becoming the wise and wild women we were born to be.

I wanted to read about journeys too, through and beyond what my soul knew to be a period in the life of a woman that elevated her to the much-misunderstood crone phase - the phase of owning our crown energy, owning our ovaries in a very different way, and to owning our sovereignty.

My desire to understand was not driven by fear, but of wanting to understand, and like I mentioned above, of wanting to succeed in my sovereignty. To not pass up this amazing opportunity to learn about this beautiful piece of creation known as the female body - a body I was blessed to journey through life with this time around.

When I approached Clarissa with the idea of collaborating with me on this book, I knew before I asked her, she would say yes.

Because our soul knows.

Always.

As the group of ladies, and one gentleman came together over the period of a year, and the chapters you will read in this book took form, the emotions within me overflowed.

The vision I had, of addressing the various cultures of nations, faiths, ethnicities, genders, generations, professions, spirituality and family all came together.

There are some cultures missing, and not because the voices were not invited, but because the voices were not ready to invest in the future generations, in the importance of their own voice, and in the healing process following years of patriarchal ruling and shaming.

Those who grace the following pages gift you some incredible insights into what it is to be a woman - and a man - travelling through the menopause in today's world.

After each chapter, you have a space to journal, reflect and interact with the energies and insights shared by each of us who said yes to the calling of our souls.

We hope you enjoy the journeys we share with you, enjoy laughing with us and that you will find what it is you are looking for.

Share the grace and goodness once you are done reading by gifting copies to those in your life, creating positive and powerful change in the world - one woman, one relationship, one family and community and one reader at a time.

If you wish to continue the conversations within these pages, reach out to us using the contact details we share with you.

With love and gratitude to you, and for you,

Dawn x

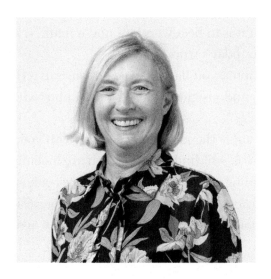

CLARISSA KRISTJANSSON
SWEDEN

Clarissa Kristjansson is an internationally recognised holistic menopause and hysterectomy coach who knows that perimenopause can be challenging but also the gateway to transformation and the emergence of a wiser woman.

In her work she supports women to develop a greater awareness of themselves, shifting their mindset on menopause from the popular narrative to become resilient, empowered, compassionate women.

She is a speaker, author of international best seller *The Mindful Menopause* and the host of the popular *Thriving Thru Menopause* podcast.

Clarissa lives with her partner and rescue dog Minnie in a small rural community on the west coast of Sweden. She is a yogi, organic gardener and has developed a passion for creating cake recipes based on vegetables.

https://clarissakristjansson.com

Chapter One

SELF-COMPASSION IN MENOPAUSE: UNLOCKING OUR PERSONAL AND COLLECTIVE FEMININE POWER

Why do some women breeze through perimenopause while others experience severe symptoms? One word: Intersectionality.

Menopause is the most significant bio-psycho-social change in a woman's life. And there is a huge array of menopausal experiences. It seems that for every woman who is struggling, there is another whose only symptom was her periods stopped. Unfortunately, we don't always have answers for these differences. But there is emerging research that indicates that some of the answers may lie in our past.

THE IMPACT OF ACES[1] ON PERIMENOPAUSE

Numerous factors influence the frequency and severity of our perimenopausal symptoms. These can include genetics, lifestyle or surgical menopause (where your ovaries are removed). Suppose we were able, to be honest with ourselves for a moment. Our lifestyle can be less than supportive of hormone balance. Skipping breakfast, endless lattes, cupcakes. Downing a bottle of wine, a night after sitting on our butts for eight to ten hours at work. Obsessively checking social media. Saying yes when no is the honest answer. Keeping our emotions

---

1   ACEs – Adverse Childhood Experiences

reined all day when you really want to scream at someone in the office. Instead, you unleash your fury on your unsuspecting child for leaving unwashed dishes in the sink. Believe me, I did that. But of all, these behaviours rarely supported us at the best of times and least of all in perimenopause.

A growing body of research demonstrates the impact of intersectionality and epigenetics on our perimenopause symptoms. One area that has obtained growing attention is Adverse Childhood Experiences or ACEs. ACEs are potentially traumatic events such as parental divorce, parental alcoholism, or witnessing violence in the home. Unfortunately, this kind of trauma is common, with two out of every three children experiencing this kind of trauma as they grow up. A situation that many women I work with, and have encountered, believe to be integral to our experiences of perimenopause.

How do ACEs cause an increase in the severity of menopausal symptoms? It is believed that toxic stress from ACEs may impact the development of the nervous system and possibly also the endocrine system. When our endocrine system is put under stress, as in perimenopause, symptoms like depression, anxiety and severe hot flashes can emerge. Sometimes these may be latently present and are triggered by the fluctuation and decline of progesterone (our soothing calming hormone) and oestrogen, which regulates the major emotional centres in the brain.

So how does knowing this help? After all, it's not like we can go back and undo the trauma. Therapy and medication can be highly effective in expanding tolerance that *may* help an individual more effectively cope with distressing perimenopause reactions. But to reduce or even remove the impact of ACEs on our perimenopause experience, we need to expand our capacity beyond enduring and coping. And that is the capacity to inhabit the body and mind with curiosity and self-compassion, which can be used to empower not only ourselves but also other women in this phase of life.

MY DESCENT INTO BECOMING AN ANXIETY SUFFERER

I had lived as an anxiety sufferer since I was eight. Until that point, I would say my childhood was as close to idyllic as is possible. I had two loving parents, loving grandmothers; I lived in a prosperous suburb of south London. And then, my life was impacted by the friction in my parents' marriage. As a child, I bore witness to the continual gaslighting of my mother. Brought on by my father's desire for separation but conflicted by his Catholic faith, led not to divorce but to devising ways to undermine her mental health and stability. Therefore, absolving him of guilt in his own twisted mind when he abandoned his family. During this dysfunctional period, his tactics included threatening to ensure my mother, a Swedish citisen, would lose her children and be deported. Foreigners could reside in Britain by marriage or the good grace of the government.

As a neuro researcher context is everything. So, my childhood situation has to be placed within the context of the prevailing status of women in the 1960s. On divorce, they had no automatic right to the marital home or custody of their children. Coupled with that, a woman required their husband's signature to obtain a mortgage or a British passport. My mother was trapped. Her choices were to live with the situation or risk losing her children. And despite approaching several law firms in search of a divorce, she could find no one willing to take on her case. So, for the intervening three years, we lived in a state of limbo, unsure what could happen next, as my father came and went as he wished. The happy extended family fell apart as sides were taken. Finally, when I turned eleven, my father announced via telephone that he was moving to Hong Kong. He disappeared except for occasional letters, always from the Kowloon courthouse where he presided over people's lives as Judge Blackwell and a few visits. In essence, I lost a parent and a family that I loved.

But it was my mother's fear and anxiety that had the most significant impact. It is hard for me to unravel how much of what she said was true or her own interpretation of events that created the rules my sister and I were made to live. Sickeningly tinged with snobbery and racism. I often wonder if in choosing an Iranian to be my first love, I was in a subtle way rebelling against her rules. The rationale was that the way we were expected to live would 'keep us safe'. School marks had to be perfect. Our family business was not to be discussed beyond the four walls of our home. So, I became an expert at lying, telling neighbours, friends, and teachers that my dad just works overseas. This, of course, he did, but not the truth that he had abandoned his family was never to be uttered.

The school years flowed on, and the rigidity of the rules meant I succeeded academically and entered university. I saw my father infrequently, and the last time was on my first day of university. His harsh critique of the course I had chosen didn't sit well, and I made the decision that I was not prepared to accept the same gaslighting as my mother had endured.

I kept my mask firmly in place through my marriage, friendships, and workplace. Consistently showing up and doing an excellent job. Yet, I had developed complex processes to ensure everything appeared perfect in the foreground. But always living with a gnawing uncertainty that someone would find out I was winging it or failing in some way. And of course, along with this approach to life came too many dysfunctional relationships, romantic and professional.

LIVING AS AN ANXIETY SUFFERER

High functioning anxiety is not a recognised mental health diagnosis. Instead, it is a catch-all term for people who live with anxiety but function well in one or more aspects of their lives. If you live with anxiety, contrary to the popular social media depiction, it can often drive you forward rather than leave you frozen in fear. Outwardly you can appear successful, together, and calm. A typical Type A personality who excels at work and life. However, on the inside, you feel very different. Beneath the surface of a seemingly calm and collected exterior, you're fighting with constant anxiety. It may manifest as nervous energy, perfectionism, and fear of disappointing others.

Someone with high functioning anxiety may display many of these characteristics. Indeed, I recognise myself in this description:

- Punctuality, arriving on time if not a bit early to work, to meetings of any nature. Impeccably dressed, not a hair out of place. I was always 10 minutes early for an appointment.
- Co-workers and bosses may say you are dedicated to your work. You deliver on the deadline and fall short in a given task. You are initiative-taking and organised – to-do lists and calendar bookings rule the day.
- In addition, you are the point of reference if someone needs help. I had no training in saying no to authority, so I acquiesced.
- You have an outgoing personality (happy, tells jokes, smiles, laughs).
- Often you appear outwardly calm and collected. I always found this the most fantastic feedback and wondered if others were blind, stupid or self-absorbed
- You are loyal in personal and professional relationships even when not serving you. Two marriages before the age of thirty-seven are the best testament to this part of me.

Despite being regarded as "high functioning," I was a "People Pleaser", afraid of driving people away, fear of being seen as a lousy friend, partner or employee, gripped by the fear of letting others down. And if others cared to be more aware, they would have seen the nervous "chatter", the nervous habits (messing with my hair, the nail-biting). The need to do repetitive things. Among my favourites was counting how many seconds it takes for the lights to change from red to green. How many steps from here to there? The overthinking, the need for reassurance, asking for directions multiple times or checking details frequently. Rumination and the endless "What if?" scenarios, as well as dwelling on past mistakes. The inability to say "No," always having an overloaded schedule, taking pride from always being busy. Although seemingly social, I could not "enjoy the moment." And a lack of natural spontaneity, choosing instead planning everything in detail, was the order of the day, even holidays.

A high-functioning person is often regarded as an overachiever. However, this perception is short-sighted because it fails to consider the struggle required to achieve that level of success. Premenopausal most people who met or knew me would not have had a clue of my day-to-day struggle. My anxiety limited my life even though I achieved success at work. I rarely did anything outside my comfort zone. I undertook activities not because I would enjoy them or expand my horizons but because they were expected of someone like myself. I learned from an early age to become adept at presenting a false persona to the world and never show my true feelings to anyone. Instead, I compartmentalised my life until, at forty-four, I became perimenopausal, and my brain-ovary- adrenal axis no longer functioned well. As a result, I couldn't process, regulate, and manage my life in the same rigid way.

PERIMENOPAUSE AND THE ANXIETY SUFFERER

My buried anxiety burst onto the surface and was visible to others. The complex rules and routines, the endless checking, list-making and inner criticism had given way to excessive nervous chatter. My biggest issue was talking over people in meetings driven by desperate anxiety that I might not be heard. The missed deadlines, the inability to focus appropriately on complex projects. For me, the worst aspect was the anxiety showed up as extreme nervousness in presentations. I was the woman who'd stood in front of big audiences of 1000's, won awards at conferences for best paper and wowed VPs with my clarity and vision. Now I couldn't manage a small webinar in somebody's office without something going wrong.

I wish I could write that my anxiety was met with empathy and understanding. But the opposite was true. Menopause is rarely discussed in the workplace, even though fifty-one per cent of us will experience this biological transition. Certainly not seventeen years ago, when there was little or no public discourse.

Like a lot of women, I couldn't disguise my symptoms. It was a sharp difference from when I was pregnant during that time; I didn't think twice about confessing forgetfulness and fatigue. Men and women laughed knowingly and supportively at my anecdotes. But in perimenopause, I was faced with blatant ageism, ableism and discrimination. And worst of all, it came from another woman. Most significantly, my direct line manager. Her vitriolic comments centred on my anxiety, making others anxious and unwilling to work for or with me. I felt crushed, but I am always minded to quote Madeleine Albright. In her keynote speech at the Celebrating Inspiration luncheon with the WNBA's All-Decade Team in 2006. As she said, "There is a special place in hell for women who don't help other women."

But there is also another obvious explanation for her outburst, as Dr Shawn Andrew outlines in her research and book *The Power of Perception (2017)*. She shows that women at higher leadership levels tend to display more male-specific EQ competencies. These appear as assertiveness and confidence. They leverage less female-specific EQ competencies, such as interpersonal relationships and empathy. My line manager displayed classic *Queen Bee Syndrome*, where women behave in ways more typical of men to demonstrate toughness and the need to fit in. Maybe I should not have been surprised. The marketing department I worked in was publicly described as having 'more testosterone than the front row of the Wallabies [2]'.

This blatant belittling also has its roots in a society where youth is over-valued. In my experience, Anglo-cultures, especially in the US and Australia, show this tendency. My peers and leaders were under forty, many unmarried, most of them childless. Perimenopause, at best, they might have asked what's that? Young was the order the day, vast amounts spent on procedures to hold back the tide of time while partying hard after work. Unsurprising, I became the outlier, the forty-seven-year-old who had to leave on time to collect her child from after school care, who could only rarely go to the after-work drinks. The

---

2   Wallabies – the mens Australian National Rugby Union team

only way I could play the game was to adopt the 'right' look. Dressing younger, dyeing my hair, Botox and filler, dating younger men. My bank balance didn't look too great as a result.

Like many workplace cultures, this organisation perpetuated patriarchy and ageism. It was intent on mining the individual's life energy to feed profits. And making it difficult for younger senior women to empathise with older women and truly support each other. My subsequent resignation was driven by anger, disappointment and betrayal. In this emotional state, I reacted to feelings rather than having a perspective on the situation. And although I was lucky to find another role. The one I was offered was less prestigious. But fear of money, a legacy of my childhood, created ridiculous unsubstantiated thoughts. This clouded the signals about the new position that was plain to see. I did not heed the messages from even the recruiter himself, who suggested I should not apply or indeed accept the role. With its supposed logical arguments, the fear overruled gut instinct and the advice of others. It became a hard lesson that was undoubtedly on my karmic path, for without it, I would never have found myself where I am today.

I joined this new organisation, and within two weeks, the consequences of my unconsidered choice were evident. First, I became acutely aware of how intense the atmosphere was within this company. Then came that pivotal moment six weeks in. It was a Friday, the first whole week of working with the newly appointed marketing director. Although I reported to him directly, he hadn't spoken to me all week. My mind was in full catastrophe mode. A series of worst-case scenarios played out in my head, but I decided to confront him. As I stepped out of the lift, he emerged from the other lift. Of course, the conversation didn't go to plan; I have no clue what I said to this day. All I can remember is feeling an out of body experience and the inability to breathe, a classic panic attack experience. He looked at me rather blankly and suggested that I take the lift rather than run up the stairs. Then turned on his heels and went into the office.

But that moment was the tipping point. With current trends in the personal development world, many of us know the phrase "the universe has your back". From the depth of my memory, I recalled a woman I had met, whose calm composure and energy had impressed itself upon me. Google is indeed our friend at such a moment. I discovered she belonged to an organisation called Openground. They train people in mindfulness. There I began a journey to building the capacity to meet and better manage my perimenopausal anxiety. Working with "brain-wise", body-based approaches. Learning to facilitate self-regulation and co-regulation. Developing an embodied sense of safety. Creating reparative relationships; and finding the ability to communicate implicit and body-based experiences.

I learned over those eight weeks the importance of awareness and that I wasn't alone in my experience of anxiety. That we are all in the same boat in this learning and growing experience we call life. Mindfulness helps us to regulate emotions through regulating attention. These are foundations for acceptance. It teaches us that rather than perpetually striving to get things lined up just right. Or reacting when things go wrong. Instead, we can learn to pause, consider and respond with thoughtful, effective action.

As I practised mindfulness, I experienced certain difficulties. I became increasingly aware of the unpleasant, painful and pleasant in each moment. This growing awareness was upsetting. It brought doubts of whether I was 'doing this right. I always thought I would feel ultimately better after embarking on this mindfulness path. But I learned that living mindfully does not mean a calm response to emotions. Instead, I learned to refrain from habitual thoughts and behaviour even though the uncomfortable feelings were still there.

Through persistent practice, mindfulness did positively impact my over-busy, overregulated self. By the end of the eight weeks of Mindfulness Based Stress Reduction (MBSR), the benefits were tangible. To a brain foggy, anxious perimenopausal woman, this was a blessing. And the sleep, ahh, a relief after the years of waking wide-eyed at 2 am. Mindfulness is, after all, about reducing suffering. So, there I was, sleeping better, eating better, committed to more exercise. I functioned closer to my old self at work and at home. And yet, mindfulness was not enough to help me turn my gnawing anxiety entirely around. Strangely despite the improvements in the way my daily life unfolded, I felt disconnected, distanced. I was still a people pleaser, unable to express my actual needs. Or take bolder steps to move life onto a footing more aligned to my personal values.

It is a natural part of meditation to feel somewhat disconnected from the outer world. As you become aware of negative emotions or obsessive thought patterns, you are motivated to retreat and draw attention inward. Each time you address a habitual pattern through awareness, you become a bit dissociated. You are unable to continue doing or believing in the same old thing. At this time, you may feel somewhat disconnected from yourself, even if what you are cutting out has clearly been a negative pattern. The Buddhist teacher Pema Chodron describes this as the 'detox period'. I didn't act on my habitual patterns, which felt more like giving up an addiction than something Zen. It is not enough for a long-term anxiety sufferer to disengage from habitual patterns. It is vital to continue to go deep inside, connect with the quality of openness, the unbounded space inside yourself, and allow warmth and creative energy to bring about personal transformation. Mindful awareness and acceptance are therefore not substitutes for deep compassion. I had to take bolder steps to heal and live well as a high anxiety sufferer and ultimately to thrive through this menopause transition and beyond.

BUT WHY COMPASSION?

A good question – why not therapy? At that point, I, like many perimenopausal women I meet, believed that therapy was admitting failure. A systemic weakness and seeking help were to be tinged with shame. So, I continued on my path. Although ultimately, I am healed and can live with my anxiety, the support of the right therapist could have gotten me there faster and more supported.

Mindfulness and compassion are often thought of as two wings of a bird in Buddhism. You need both to fly. We're training our minds to notice what's happening and regard it with compassion. The difference is what we're emphasising. The psychologist Christopher Germer (2009) explains the difference as compassion regulating difficult emotions through care and connection. While mindfulness is about bringing awareness and clarity to our habitual patterns so you can feel moments of calm and reflection. Personally, I would say that mindfulness gives us the skills and stability of mind to help us build our self-compassion. Practising self-compassion and compassion for others can bring strong feelings, including sadness, grief, anger, guilt and shame. We need a strong, calm base to work with our emotions.

Equanimity[3], kindness, and compassion are present in all of us, and are the elements of our most profound human nature. Practising mindfulness helped me recognise my patterns of behaviour and my habits. Yet, I had not learnt how to respond to these with kindness and compassion. Nor how to remain present in intense anxiety situations. I needed to cultivate an even-mindedness or composure in the face of stress.

The meditation teacher Jack Kornfield says that equanimity develops in us as we learn to keep our hearts open through the changing circumstances of our life. That felt appropriate as menopause requires a unique strength and willingness to stay present. This is not avoidance, willpower over or enduring our symptoms. Rather it is an act of bringing careful and open-hearted attention to what is here. Not turning away but softening into what is present, accepting things as they are in this moment, even if that means we must be open to unpleasant experiences. If we can do that with our menopause symptoms, we discover that what is already in us is the ability to be composed. We are unshakable.

Understanding and working in this way helps us see through compassion's misconception. It is just being kind or sympathetic. In my personal experience, believing that it is about self-care and sympathy is an over-simplification of the power of compassion. It isn't weak, emotive, or letting you off the hook. Unfortunately, too many of us believe the misconception that if you practice self-compassion, you'll be OK, and your anxiety will evaporate. Nor is compassion about trying to sweep

---

3   Equanimity – Mental calmness, composure and self-assurance

things under the carpet or soothe yourself with good external things, as in the popular self-care narratives that inundate our social feeds. Instead, sometimes it's about giving us the courage to confront who we are and our perimenopause journey with kindness. The kindness to face our anxieties, meet our physical, mental and emotional difficulties, and find peace. For myself and other women going through perimenopause, compassion can unlock the wisdom within each of us. So, we can move into Cronedom. This wisdom is empowered and empowering. Not just for ourselves but for other women too.

MY JOURNEY TO BECOMING A COMPASSIONATE SELF

I would love to be able to say that my journey into compassion was deliberate and planned, but that would be a lie. Instead, I fell, or rather, I was pushed to attend a workshop with a visiting British organisation called Breathworks. It was the beginning of the journey to complete the missing part that mindfulness couldn't provide. By 2015 I was on the last leg of the teacher training program. It was a languid afternoon, the kind you get in the South of Sydney in the middle of February, where the heat hangs and your energy feels sapped. We were sitting in the small library at the Vijyaloka retreat centre, seeking refuge from the heat of the afternoon. My mentor Karen and I reviewed my reflection diaries when she turned to me and asked, "Did you forget to do that compassion part of the training?"

"What do you mean?" I asked.

"Did you rush through this part of the coursework, or did you just forget about it or maybe you didn't understand what was required?" She questioned again.

I felt annoyance, a constriction in my chest and underneath the fear. Fear that I'd somehow failed, that I had been found out for not being good enough. No, I did that work, I said somewhat defensively. But the anxiety was palpable, that I wasn't fit to be a mindfulness practitioner, that I was going to fail. Since the first training, the feeling had lingered that I wasn't liked and didn't live up to the required standards.

Luckily, Karen is compassion personified beneath her wild Irishness.

I have always loved how loud and how much she swears with her students. Working with her and listening rather than just showing up provided me with a better understanding of the concept of becoming a compassionate self. Someone who has the wisdom to know that we didn't choose the root of our suffering. But that we can be motivated to learn, grow and change. That inside each of us, there is inner confidence and strength that can emerge from that wisdom. We can develop and learn to take responsibility to not run away from our problems through open friendliness. Instead, we commit to working and act in ways that are helpful to ourselves.

To further support my journey, Karen directed me to the teachings of psychologist Christopher Germer and the Buddhist teacher Tara Brach. Germer's *The Mindful Path to Self-Compassion* became my constant companion. I began to spend my lunchtime in the Sydney Botanical Gardens reading and absorbing this simple wisdom. Brach's R-A-I-N practice has become a pillar for my own life and for my work with my clients. It is a way of engaging with our experience and investigating. Hence, it becomes workable and a source of knowledge and wisdom. Brach's "little acronym" RAIN moves through four steps.

R – Recognising and honouring rather than avoiding difficult emotions. Perimenopause is often filled with avoidances. We may deny our symptoms or the role of intersectionality instead of blaming the hormones for every ill. But turning to see, feel and know our painful experiences open us to a new way of thriving in menopause.

A – Allowing our difficulties to be here. Giving ourselves space to 'be with' rather than problem-solving or taking the quick fix has become synonymous with perimenopause.

I – Investigating the body, the emotions, the thoughts, the stories that arise at this moment. I find this of immense value for addressing perimenopause, where negativity and an over-emphasis on the twenty per cent who experience a difficult menopause journey have become the blueprint for everyone. Here we examine our own narratives and expectations. How we can gain insight into these patterned responses and question their validity within the context of our own experience.

N – Non-identifying with what is arising. This is liberation. Stepping back and seeing your experience as phenomena of shifting sensations, emotions and narratives in the process of being generated, staying around a while and then changing. Seeing your experience like weather passing through a vast and spacious sky. Non-identification in perimenopause can help with over-identification with our symptoms and begins to give us space to see what underlies or fuels our anxiety, our pain beyond the physiological. It can help us to see that all who reside in a female body in perimenopause are in a similar boar. We all suffer. We can grow to know our pain and patterns and open up to how to respond in each moment.

These meditations unexpectedly brought up despair, shame, failure and rage. But when I stopped fighting them and started feeling them, my relationship with my anxiety shifted. When prompted to examine where feelings lived in my body. Anger and fear manifested as tension in the jaw, shoulders, and chest. Nurturing was usually the most difficult and the most powerful. When I put my hands on the heart or wrapped myself in a hug and whispered aloud, "It's OK, you are OK." The practice helped me understand my situation and started healing from the pain I had lived with for so long.

My own experience is that compassion practices are visceral. Compassion has given me the ability to be with the roots of my anxiety. It impacted my perimenopause and unfolded into a warm and connected process where I was able to heal through coming into a new relationship with myself, and later through connection and deeper relationships with others.

Cultivating compassion over time has brought me an intuitive, immediate and relational way of living. And finding a place where all of me is welcome. Too often, I had felt 'on show', the need to be seen as high achieving and successful. While on the inside, loneliness and shame and the desire sometimes to be in oblivion were suppressed, even though these are natural human experiences. Compassion taught me not to identify so strongly with my anxiety to the point that it limited my sense of self. Instead, I could take the step to give over to listening to the many parts of me that were often contradictory and call upon a generous spirit and deep permission to be here, known and healed. That my anxiety could have the care and attention rather than my aversion and contempt. And that discovering my inner resources allowed the beauty inside me to be discovered. That my perimenopausal symptoms could be given compassionate, courageous, spacious presence. And that through curiosity, care and love, I could allow them to be here, listening, allowing space and freedom and a platform to start healing. From this place, I could make compassionate choices.

And it is precisely these choices that have the most powerful impact when it comes to your health and, healing the ones that are your own. These have the most powerful impact on your body, on your soul, on your sense of self. For me, these choices manifested as values by which I have chosen to live my life and habits that support these values. And they have become non-negotiables, and my life feels more vibrant and purposeful as a result. In formulating these, I have been greatly inspired by the work of Caroline Myss in the fields of human consciousness, spirituality and mysticism, health, energy medicine, and the science of medical intuition.

I choose not to pass on my perimenopause drama. We all have pain and grief but need to keep sharing it. I decided not to over-identify with it. It's not about denying the difficulties but learning from them and choosing to share the wisdom that those experiences have given me and can support others going through this life transition.

I choose to take calculated risks. As Myss says in one of her reflections, we must never look backwards for guidance . We weaken ourselves by continually looking backwards, and instead, we can embrace the "newness" of possibility. Don't ask for everything to be easy. Stop searching for a quick fix. Refuse to slide into regretful living.

I choose a positive language. If your words are toxic, your vocabulary is fundamentally hostile toward everyone and, most importantly, yourself. It perpetuates the internal dialogue that perimenopause is hard. The inner criticism that you see your life as not enough. You see others as not enough. Your first reaction to everything is critical. As we move through the peri to post-menopause journey, I invite you to avoid words that promote those thoughts or reactions. Myss strongly suggests we avoid three powerful words: 1) blame, 2) deserve, 3) entitled; and that to extricate these words from our head would enable us to feel so much better.

I choose to get up and bless my day. And don't base your gratitude for your life on what you have or how you feel. The fantastic thing about gratitude is that it doesn't have to be about the big stuff for you to feel the benefits. Gratitude can shape the life around you with grace and beauty. Even when perimenopause symptoms are hard to bear, being present with great gratitude supports us.

Learning to live this way empowered me through the remaining time of my perimenopause and into this next stage of life. The one that Asian cultures so aptly have named the *Second Spring*. Through this experience of becoming a compassionate self, I also see the power that compassion has to support other women. Not just to change their individual experiences but as a platform for creating inclusive change in the world. This is where my journey has taken a new direction. To champion a greater, more inclusive empowerment of women. Harnessing the energy that the menopause transformation awakens and how we can use this to drive a more inclusive empowering experience for ourselves and the generations who will follow us.

EMPOWERING OUR MENOPAUSE AND OUR COLLECTIVE FEMININE POWER

Once I began to love myself, it triggered me to start asking questions about menopausal women, how they were, and their place in the world. Compassion can become a steppingstone to questioning and changing our cultural views of the peri to post-menopause transition. In valuing ourselves, I, like many other women, have become overly aware of how much our culture drives reinforcement of outdated cultural norms that display a notable lack of humanity.

Imagine that we discovered a new condition that would affect roughly half the population. It would involve some of the following in varying degrees and combinations: cardiovascular disease, osteoporosis, neurological symptoms, Alzheimer's disease, joint pain, and decreased sex drive. In addition, the problems associated with perimenopause can last for ten years or more to compound this. Yet, unlike COVID, we are not throwing billions of dollars of government funding trying to sort it out. Even though this is a condition that affects all women at some stage of their lives (and men!).

In the 19th century, menopause was associated with 'moral insanity demonstrated by peevishness and fits of temper or self-absorption and exacerbated by reading novels, dancing, or going to the theatre'. Unfortunately, today not nearly enough has changed. Thankfully, we are now taking mental health and gender identity and equality seriously, in addition to physical health. By extension, we really should take the experience of menopause transition more seriously.

Historically and traditionally, women's bodies have been a transactional tool to please men or for their biological functions. For many women, sexuality, desirability, attractiveness, and functionality as a child-bearer are elements of how others perceive and value you. Sociocultural theorists describe how the Western media subjects women to unrelenting pressure to conform to a largely unachievable body ideal. Even though this is portrayed as easily obtainable and leads to body dissatisfaction across the lifespan. However, self-compassion can change the way women, particularly older women seen by society as less valuable, show up in our male-dominated world. Too often, we are taught to view ourselves with self-criticism, with the urge to change the essence of who we are or to preferably fade into anonymity. This is has led women into situations in which they falsely believe that self-improvement rather than self-compassion is the key.

Additionally, objectification theory emphasises how women are taught to view their bodies as outside observers from an early age. This body surveillance leads to shame when they do not meet such culturally constructed ideas of femininity. And it is the silence that this shame and stigma bring that is the real enemy. In Western society, older women are praised for retaining youthful looks and countering the biological tendency to gain weight. Media aimed specifically at women in their forties and fifties reflects this. Menopause commonly occurs when women's appearances depart from Western cultural beauty ideals of youth and thinness.

The feminist discourse emphasises that menopause can be a positive or neutral change. But this is difficult when women are bombarded with a predominant biomedical discourse that treats menopause as a series of biological and physiological deficiencies and changes, which require treatment and damage the underlying truth. That the peri to post-menopause time is a natural and profound transformation.

Concurrently, media treatments of menopause promote the idea that women can remain the same as they have always been. These narratives legitimise women's fears that they are of little value if they change. These stories benefit multiple industries. Recent analysis valued the global skincare market at US$134.8 billion with increased demand for anti-ageing products, one of the key factors boosting industry growth. This has been further fuelled by the development and growth of 'menopause' skincare, something I detest. In Britain alone, the beauty industry's contribution to GDP was almost £24.8 billion in 2018, more than the motor vehicle manufacturing or publishing industries. And that is further compounded by probably the most toxic industry – the diet industry.

The global market for weight loss products and services in 2021 is valued at $255 billion. It is forecasted to reach $377.3 billion by 2026, at a compound annual growth rate of 8.2 per cent during the forecast period of 2021-2026. $10 billion of which can be attributed to directly targeting menopausal women. Even though certified nutritionists are clear that traditional dieting and weight-loss strategies have negligible impact on that 'meno-belly'. In fact, most of us will have a softer, rounder body, and weight per se is a poor measure of our health as we age. Stop fighting your body. Instead, celebrate the gifts you have to give, value your body and its wisdom.

But as long as we take things the way they are, we stay complicit in the shame, the stigma and the silence surrounding the female cycle in its entirety. Living this way, we're perpetuating that we are unworthy of abundance. That we are incapable of self-regulation and require medication to survive perimenopause. The debate is currently very focused on HRT as the solution, which can undoubtedly improve the quality of women's lives but increasingly is sold as a panacea for hormonal imbalances. In so doing, we downgrade the conversation about intersectionality, leaving many to having what can be described as 'menopause on the margins'.

Suppose we bring compassion to the conversation to create a social shift, the discussion needs to also include how the structure of our economy intends to prey on women's feelings of not being good enough. Like racism and sexism, discrimination based on age serves a social and economic purpose: to legitimise and sustain inequalities. It's less about how we look. And more about how people in power assign meaning to how we look. Unless we challenge ageist stereotypes: that older women are incompetent, wrinkles are ugly, and it's sad to be old, we will continue to feel shame and embarrassment instead of taking pride in accomplishing our first fifty or so years on this earth. Then we internalise ageism. And as the debate on menopause opens up, we can see that vast swathe of the industries. The coaching world, beauty industry and the health and fitness industry are built on reinforcing how bad or inadequate we are as we age. And how much we need rescuing from a natural part of life. Those who choose not to take HRT are shamed on social media. Influencers drive a narrative that everyone MUST demand from her clinician HRT. If the doctor refuses HRT on medical grounds or is not on the latest research, they are too vilified.

You might say that menopause is 'having a moment'. Since the beginning of 2021, the debate on menopause has become more elevated. We are beginning to challenge these cultural norms individually and collectively. We are awakening to questions: Why are the society and economy still holding onto this patriarchal approach to living? Who are we now? What is our role in society? What is our value? These questions need to be reflected upon and from which policies should be developed. A fascinating recent Australian research paper titled *Killer*

Whales and Killer Women suggests that leadership is an innate gift that postmenopausal women possess (Krajewski, 2019). One that we have acquired by midlife through our experiences and that enables many of us to step into leadership roles on a local, community, national or international levels.

An under-explored aspect of self-compassion relates to power in the world. There's a strong connection between loving yourself and directing resources globally. Power is the ability to get things done and direct resources towards accomplishing a particular goal. And fierce self-compassion helps us hold a powerful centre. It can support us make our dreams a reality, advocating for justice or doing whatever work we are called to do. When self-compassion is present, you know your own preferences and desires. It's not that you're always putting yourself first; you also know your limits and capacities and when you can go that extra mile. Your boundaries might be narrow or broad and all-encompassing, but you know what they are. So, in your wider work, you're able to take the steps needed to take care of yourself or let yourself be cared for.

If you wish to move things in a particular direction, self-compassion gives you a strong, stable foundation of your own, with real clarity about what you want to accomplish. If you're less likely to be leaning out into what other people need and moving away from your own stable base, it's challenging to have any leverage in outside action. Self-compassion helps you stay in your own core and act from a place of strength and stability. That's one piece of the "power" component.

Power is how we internalise what society believes about our own worth. If we lack fierce self-love, there is a greater chance that we won't even stand up for our own values or those of others. This behaviour can be so deeply internalised that we denigrate our self-worth and are unable to advocate for ourselves or for other menopausal women as was so plainly demonstrated by my line manager. It also shows up regularly in the press, where journalists take the stance that women are moaning about their symptoms and should 'Suck it up, buttercup'.

So self-compassion isn't, therefore, only the yin version popularised on social media where bubble baths and indulgence, fantastic as they are, that centre stage. Instead, compassion is that perfect blend of yin and yang. The concept of yang or fierce compassion was first championed by Kristin Neff (2020) as part of the broader #MeToo discourse. That it's not just tender self-compassion, we need to get through the mess of menopause. We also need fierce self-compassion. In other words, we don't want to just be complacent about this stage in life. We also want to do what we can to change things for the better, inside ourselves and outside of us. Part of fierce self-compassion is fighting for justice, drawing boundaries, motivating change. This is also an essential part of compassion as we wade through the mess of menopause. It is where self-love becomes about essential-ness, the essence of who we are that we are worthy, creative beings who, through greater perspective, have choices. That's when self-compassion ripples out beyond ourselves, our closest relationships and into creating a just, more equal culture.

For those in perimenopause that means that no one can dissuade you from the fact that you deserve equal health care. Equal pay and the right to work without being discriminated against based on age or symptoms. Stand in your own power and bring compassion to your own being. Because from that you can do remarkable things in the world. While we're internalising a new reverence for ourselves, we're also solving systemic problems that stem from a lack of respect for the feminine. We have started to champion the need for dignified menopause. One where our most significant life transition is honoured and celebrated. You are seen as a whole person, and menopause is not demoted to a series of physiological events to be diagnosed and treated. Consciousness-raising, like those used in the civil rights movements of the US, are essential to the process of social change that involves conversation, collaboration, activism, art, advocacy, and eventually legislation.

As we learn to take care of our own being, it is compelling us to write a new story, that of inclusive menopause. Despite the elevated dialogue, the narrative remains largely Anglo, white, heterosexual and middle class. Though the conversation has to start somewhere, for all of us to have dignified menopause, we need to dismantle existing menopause stereotypes. Raising the awareness of diverse menopause experiences and supporting that menopause materials are inclusive of people's needs. I have been personally honoured to be part of the Global Menopause Inclusion Collective, a collaboration of menopause activists, advocates, experts by experience, researchers, individuals and professionals interested in advancing equality, equity, diversity and inclusion in the menopause movement. Working together in this way, we can challenge traditional views of menopause. Changing the way we talk about menopause embraces our full life experiences as menstruators. Irrespective of our race, ethnicity, age, gender identity, disability or socioeconomic status, instead of creating a more compassionate, inclusive society that becomes the rewriting of the menopause story for all of us. And that's true power.

REFERENCES

Andrews, S. (2017) Power of Perception: Leadership, Emotional intelligence, and the gender divide. New York: Morgan James Publishing.

Germer, C. (2009) The Mindful Path to Self-Compassion – Freeing yourself from destructive thoughts and emotions. New York: The Guilford Press.

Krajewski, S. (2019) Killer Whales and Killer Women: Exploring menopause as a "Satellite Taboo" that orbits madness and old age, in Sexuality and Culture, 23, 605-620. https://doi.org/10.1007/s12119-018-9578-3

Neff, Kristin (2020) Fierce Self-Compassion, mindfulness and the #MeToo Movement. (https://www.mindfulnessbasedcoach.com/blog/2019/10/29/fierce-self-compassion-mindfulness-and-the-metoo-movement)"

Reflections

Reflections

Reflections

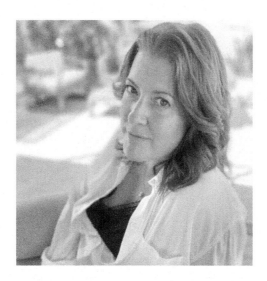

DAWN BATES
LOCATION-FREE

Dawn Bates is a true international bestselling author multiple times over on five continents. She specialises in developing authorities who wish to give a voice to the voiceless whilst guiding them to create brand expansion strategies through activism, authorship and business.

With social justice and human rights underpinning everything she does, including her study with the University of Oxford where she is working towards her PhD in Human Rights and Social Justice, you can guarantee her books are powerful.

Dawn brings together the multi-faceted aspects of the world we live in and takes you on a rollercoaster ride of emotions, whilst delivering mic dropping inspiration, motivation and awakening. Her work captures life around the world in all its rawness.

To discover more about Dawn, please visit www.dawnbates.com

For all those wishing to regain some focus and take the next steps towards a more empowered future, make sure you check out and sign up for Dawn's *21 Day Phoenix UpRising Lifestyle Reboot* using this special offer code: **menopause**

Chapter Two

MAMA NEVER TOLD ME

Having the desire to eat chocolate like I had never had before, I headed out into the garden to get my bike so I could go to the village shop and get the biggest bar of chocolate my piggy bank would allow.

My bike had a flat tyre and the desire for chocolate was overwhelming, so I took my brothers racing bike. Half way to the shop, a car backed out of the driveway and as I pulled the brakes, I was thrown forward landing on the crossbar of the bike.

The pain was excruciating and hot tears stung my eyes, but the desire for chocolate won hands down, so I continued to the shop as fast as I could.

As soon as I arrived home and had put my brother's bike back in the garage, I headed straight to the toilet, because now the desire to go to the toilet was larger than the 1kg bar of Cadbury's whole nut chocolate I had just purchased.

I felt this immense ache and this urge to pee, and a sensation I had never felt before, like something was being pulled out of my uterus. Not that I knew what the word uterus was, or why my left leg ached so much.

Sitting on the toilet my pee sounded different, and it felt different coming out of me. When I looked down and saw all the blood on the inside of my legs and in the toilet, I screamed to my mum. "Mum!! I've cut myself! There's blood everywhere!" My mum came running from the kitchen where she was preparing dinner for when Dad came home later that evening. "Look Mum! I'm bleeding!"

Taking a quick look my mum said, "You've not cut yourself; you've started your periods. Now get yourself cleaned up, put one of these in your knickers. Then you've got your homework to get done".

"But Mum…" I started.

"Don't 'But Mum' me, you were always going to be an early starter. You'll probably start the menopause early too, but don't ask me what to expect with that, I won't know because I've had a hysterectomy so won't get it. Now I have to put dinner in the oven ready for when your dad gets home. And don't eat all that chocolate before dinner… but bring it with you and we'll have some together with a cuppa tea".

Early starter? Menopause? Hysterectomy? Words my nine-year-old brain just didn't know about, and how the heck did Mum know to give me one of these pads to put in my knickers before she had even arrived in the toilet?

So, over our cup of tea and a quarter of the bar of chocolate each, I asked her, "Mum, how did you know I had started my periods? And what is a hysterectomy? And what is menopause?"

"You've been getting all emotional and snappy. Your boobs have started budding and you have been wanting chocolate. Your periods are the start of your journey to being able to have babies" and with the warning tone in her voice and a half smile - half stern look on her face she continued with "which you even think about having until you're at least twenty-five and with someone worthy of being a dad, I'll come down on you like a tonne of bricks young lady"

"I won't have a baby until I am at least married and have my own business" I told her, to which she responded "Hmmm I don't disbelieve you. Anyway, hysterectomy is where they whip out your bits, like they did mine after I had your sister so I can't get pregnant again, and the menopause is where your periods stop and you are supposed to get all hot, sweaty and even more miserable than when you are on a period".

"I am going to get all hot, sweaty and miserable on a period?" I asked.

"Depends. Knowing how you just sped off to get chocolate, you'll probably want chocolate a few days before your period starts too. The same goes for the menopause, and I said, '*you are supposed to*', but knowing you, you'll do things differently. It's different for everyone. When you have finished the menopause at around sixty, that's when your periods will stop too; but like I said, I haven't had the menopause so don't know much about it. I won't have it either. Now here, put these in your school bag, and keep these in the bathroom. Always keep one with you when you are on your period or about due, and then you will never be caught short".

This was the introduction to the rest of my life as a 'woman' – a female of child bearing age, one who was destined to eat chocolate, be hot, moody and sweaty for at least a week every month until I had finished the menopause. 'Welcome to the next fifty years of life as a woman' I thought to myself.

I went up to my room to do my homework but walking up the wooden hill as my dad called it, my homework changed from maths and geography to "What is menopause?". Looking through the encyclopaedia of biology, I saw the menopause was for really old ladies like my Nan who wore slacks and an apron, had her hair set, did their knitting and baked jam tarts. I had a long way to go, so I closed the book and never gave much thought to the menopause again, other than the brief mentions it was given in the biology lessons in my senior years at school – which I could have written on the back of a postage stamp.

That was until my friend Ali recommended the book *The Red Tent* by Anita Diamant (1997) to me when I was twenty-eight. In this fictional tale describing a community of women who bled together and shared stories, I learnt so much about women and their flow – and I had this overwhelming sense of loss and grief. Where was my community? Where was my mother's community? I had never seen or experienced such a community and didn't even know of one.

I called my mum and asked her about when she didn't have such a community, and her response shocked me, "If you can count your friends on more than one hand by the time you are thirty, then you've done alright." I had just over a year to go, and as far as I was concerned, I was one of the luckiest women on the planet, because I would need more arms and legs to count my friends!

The loss and grief subsided but a lingering 'something' remained, and I didn't know what it was, but I knew there was something missing, knowledge, intimacy, connection… something I couldn't quite put my finger on. I didn't know what it was, and there was no business plan to guide me to it. So, I just allowed this missing something to present itself to me

I didn't have to wait long because shortly after the birth of my second and final child at the age of twenty-nine, I had time to just sit and think, or rather lie there and think as I had faced my own mortality due to experiencing HELLP Syndrome[1]. Having time to just lie in a hospital bed rethinking my life, what I wanted to achieve, the kind of mother I wanted to be and whether I wanted to continue with the businesses my husband and I had created together or sell it. I needed to figure out what I wanted out of life, what kind of legacy I wanted to create and, as I lay there in hospital so many things came to the forefront.

I got present to what my mum meant about the friends being counted on one hand. I realised many of the people I saw as friends were simply party friends or business colleagues – and not the kind of people I could reply on to take care of my children or show up to help when I needed it. Many were not the kind of people I wanted to share personal goals,

---

1   Hemolysis, Elevated Liver enzymes and Low Platelets–HELLP Syndrome – a condition where your body starts to shut down and abort your baby to keep you alive. https://www.preeclampsia.org/hellp-syndrome

wins or my deepest fears with. They had already proven they were not the kind of people who had celebrated and encouraged me up to this point in life, so why bother continuing with them in my life? Looking at my life, the female friends I knew I could rely on were Ali, my friend who had recommended The Red Tent, my feisty Scottish friend Amira, and Debbie – the friend I never argued with and the one who had rushed me to the hospital when the HELLP symptoms really kicked in.

Lying in hospital I knew I had to make profound changes in my life, and the first substantial change would be my husband and I moving to Egypt with our two sons so we could be closer to our family there, and in Lebanon. Leaving the UK was a big step and little did I know this thirty-third year of my life would change the trajectory of my life immeasurably or reintroduce me to 'The Menopause'.

My mother-in-law was a formidable woman, and not someone to make an enemy of. She was feared and disliked, yet highly respected and loved by all the women in her family. She didn't have many friends and neither did she want them. She had her sisters and her cousins and even though there was discontent in the ranks with her being the fierce matriarch, when they got together, they shared their journey of womanhood with each other.

I would sit and listen, seeing a bond between these women I never saw when our husbands or other men were around. They discussed how their menfolk would frustrate the hell out of them and how even in the heat of the Egyptian sun nothing compared to the furnace of their own bodies. Copious amounts of camomile tea were enjoyed and afternoon naps were highly recommended. There was a knowing between them and I was told one day I would find out for sure what they were all talking about.

After four years in Egypt during the Uprising, my children and I returned to the UK, with my divorce becoming final just six months later. My eighteen-year marriage was over and I had to dig deep and rediscover the kind of woman and mother I wanted to be and had to be. I was luckier than some because I was able to hit the ground running having had years of running my own businesses, mentoring and coaching other entrepreneurs and leaders, whilst juggling board positions, community projects, lone parenting and open house gatherings.

I dived into healing my pain and came across womb healing, which led me to cord cuttings, ancestral healing and yoni eggs. My mum had divorced my father when I was four, my sister was divorced and now I was divorced. I was seeing a pattern and knew there was definitely ancestral healing which was needed to break this pattern. Seeing the yoni eggs, my mind flashed back to the bowls of crystal eggs in the home of every Egyptian household.

I was confused. Why would yoni eggs be in bowls in the lounges of Arabian women and used as decorative centre pieces? Was it to be around the healing energies? Were these women even aware of the power of these eggs? Did they know they should have them but had a piece of the ancient wisdom puzzle missing? So many questions I wanted to ask but now I was no longer a part of the family, I had no one to ask, and no one I felt I could turn to and journey with through my own menopause when it finally arrived.

The closer I got to my fortieth birthday the more my future started to occupy my mind, and for someone who was always creating her vision of the future and thinking about how to be the best version of self, not just for me but as a role model for my boys, this is saying something.

I had been in a relationship for eighteen months and was beginning to realise it was toxic and needed to end. My new business was starting to take off, and a reoccurring dream I'd had since was a young girl returned. The dream consisted of me walking along the cliff edges with my dogs back to a stone cottage which had a jetty below with my boat tied up to it. No man beside me, no children with me, just me and my dogs.

Was this my future, a woman alone facing the wild winds of the world with just my dogs for company? Was this the future I wanted, or did I want to spend my life with someone? I had a lot of soul searching to do, but first I had to focus on the matters at hand, such as fighting the court case in Scotland which should never have happened[2].

One night a friend turned up at my home with a bottle of wine and told me I was to take a break from studying the law and working on my business. As we chatted, she mentioned she had been to see the doctor because she was in need of HRT. "HRT? Really? Why?" was my response. "Because of the menopause. I am exhausted all the time, and hungry like you wouldn't believe! I keep losing focus, forgetting what I was doing, and it's like... well like being pregnant without the baby. It's a fucking nightmare!"

As we ordered dinner she asked for tofu. I looked at her confused "Tofu? Why are you ordering tofu when you were a red bloodied meat eater?" She started telling me she had recently given up meat and all animal products and the reason she had gone vegan and started eating lots of tofu was because women in China didn't get the menopause because of the amount of tofu they ate. She wanted to avoid the menacing menopause, so was preparing herself in the perimenopause stage – hence the HRT.

My mind was racing. Preparing for menopause? And really? Tofu stopped the menopause!? I couldn't stand tofu! And HRT? I thought that was to do with the thyroid! And why was she so worried about menopause? She had years to go yet! But apparently not, she was already in the initial stages of menopause, which isn't menopause, and is why she had gained weight, needed extra B6 and B12, and was a moody cow all the time.

"But I thought we didn't get the menopause until we were like... "I started laughing "Oh my days! I was just about to say really old! We're not old, and the menopause happens to old women, retired women like our nans".

"Yeah well, brace yourself," she said, "Perimenopause is a bitch."

After she had left my mind was racing with confusion, mostly still stuck on the thought of having to eat tofu to prevent the menopause.

---

2   Detailed in my third book Crossing the Line
https://dawnbates.com/crossingtheline

I was also slightly annoyed at myself for not having taken the time to learn more about the menopause. I was always prepared, I was the one that did all the research, had all the answers to the questions my friends needed. I was the geek, the one who went down every rabbit hole looking for answers. So why did I not know about what to really expect during menopause? Why had I side stepped it? Was it simply because I thought I had at least twenty years to go before it happened?

And why was there no information on it when I had been researching the womb healing? THAT annoyed me.

I called my mum at home. I needed to talk with her. I wanted answers as to whether she had noticed any changes in her body after having a hysterectomy. Surely, she must have had some symptoms of having some kind of menopause! She said she'd had a few hot flushes a few years after her hysterectomy, but nothing she could directly say was menopause "It's just life, and you just get on with it" was her conclusion; the matter of fact, no nonsense way of looking at life.

My dad was in the background teasing me about God help the world when the hot sweats and mood swings started with me. I was already hot headed, moody on a period and ate more chocolate in the space of two days than most people ate in a lifetime. Laughter ensued between us all because eating a packet of peanut M&M's and a trio of Lindt chocolate balls was not a huge amount of chocolate! Hot headed yes, moody ... er... well... yes... I could be, but only when people were stupid and got in my way.

I mean who walks along the middle of the pavement slower than a dead person and doesn't realise that the rest of us have to get somewhere? I mean seriously!? And the people who would just stop in the middle of the street – like are you for real? And then there were the people who ate noisily with their mouth open – disgusting! And don't even get me started on people who wrapped their kids up in cotton wool and said their children were their best friends! Oh, I could get off on a rant and debate with the political leaders of the day – and had done at many a political husting, a regional regeneration event, and in the studios of radio and tv stations.

Were these rants part of the menopause? Surely not. I had been ranting and raving (including the musical kind) on many occasions throughout my life.

Was I getting hot sweats and not noticing it because I worked out and danced about the house so much?

Was I eating more chocolate that usual? Was I getting cravings for certain kinds of food? I started to 'keep watch' on the foods I ate, how I felt after them and upped the detoxes I was doing to remove certain food groups to see how my body reacted when they were reintroduced, just like I had some ten years earlier (before it was trendy).

It was time to get prepared and really investigate this menopause malarky and get to the bottom of it, because as I had always said "Poor performance is a result of piss poor planning" so I had better get on with researching so I could plan my menopause. I had things to do, and nothing was going to stop me – including the menopause.

I started looking for books in the local library whilst researching human rights, criminal and family law. The looks on the faces of the librarians was priceless – especially one chap who asked me if my menopause was that bad, I had murdered my entire family and was figuring out how to best defend myself.

Although I laughed at the humour, I was beginning to realise that most people were of the assumption that when women hit the menopause, it was time to brace themselves and prepare for an onslaught of angry abuse, emotional breakdowns and lots of chocolate eating.

What was it with the chocolate? Not that I minded. I had upgraded from the milk chocolate Lindt balls to the dark chocolate ones and anything less than 87per cent dark chocolate just wasn't worth bothering with, unless it was the white chocolate chunks in the cranberry's cookies from McVities which I would devour when I sat down long enough to watch a Sunday movie with my boys.

I started my hap hazard research into menopause and I discovered that divorce was higher within couples during the menopause years and having just gone through my divorce I momentarily wondered if my now ex-husband had made his exit on the fast track out of the marriage before menopause hit. A thought that was dismissed immediately but it did leave me wondering how many men did walk out instead of leaning in to support women through what was turning out to be a ghastly time of life.

The books in the library on menopause were clinical, boring and were more focused on the biological changes which would happen. There was no determining age, more of an age bracket which was as useful as the five hour time frames given by utility companies coming to fix something in the home. The list of possible 'conditions' was long, and yet nothing was definite. Everything listed *might happen*, but we must *prepare for all eventualities* something I was great at... but oh my lady was the future bleak!

With all the depressing news about the up-and-coming events of my future as a woman, I distracted myself with the human rights abuses around the world and continued preparing for the court case in The Scotland Saga[3] - but still that seed of eternal misery as a woman had been planted.

I didn't give it water, nor did I give it sunshine, I just let it sit there in the recesses of my mind waiting for the right time to deal with it – which came a few years later at the age of forty-one when another female friend got really aggressive with me for no reason and then blamed it on perimenopause. What the hell was this perimenopause!? This was now the second time I had heard about it, but not read about it. Was that the spicy version of menopause? The Portuguese version? The only peri I knew about was peri-peri sauce on the chicken at Nando's! So, with a pen and notepad at the ready I listed all I knew, which was the following:

- Periods stopped with the menopause, saving on cramps and a small fortune in sanitary protection – and the planet
- Women ate more chocolate than normal, but regardless of this they gained weight

---

3   The Scotland Saga is the name given to the story of my illegal detention and kidnapping of my children by Police Scotland which I mentioned above in relation to my third book *Crossing the Line*

- We would need HRT to keep our thyroid in check and our hormones
- We must eat more tofu and preferably go vegan
- Hot sweats, mood swings were the order of the day
- Others walking on egg shells were also on the order otherwise attempted murder was possible
- It wasn't just old grannies who knitted and baked jam tarts who got the menopause
- Divorce rates increased during the menopausal years
- Children were no longer possible
- If you have had a hysterectomy, you knew nothing about the menopause
- Life was over so best look for a rubbish heap to go and place ourselves on

Writing down this list, I laughed because I remembered what my mum had told me the day I started my periods "Knowing you, you'll do it differently". Then a thought occurred to me: If I had started my periods early, was I likely to start the menopause early? Did it matter what age you started your periods as to when you would start the menopause?

My plan to research and prepare for menopause has taken more side steps than an American doing the line dance, and before I knew it, I was heading to my forty-second birthday. Very little research had been done on the subject of menopause, and I realised I had simply got to the point of being even more like my mother and resigning myself to "What happens, happens. No point in worrying about it", and no offence to my mother, but that just wasn't me. I had to be prepared. I had to ace this menopause, and anything less than a ninety per cent pass rate was a fail.

So far, I had found out there were three stages of menopause: The hot and spicy perimenopause, full blown menopause (whatever form that took) and post menopause which my inner witch was telling me would be the most beautiful and liberating time in my life. The awakening of The Crone, our years of wisdom which we would boldly pass onto the younger generations and it was this stage I was really looking forward to.

Thinking back through my life, I started to connect the dots of my inner wise witch and this deep sense of knowing that this age of menopause was something to look forward to. Then I remembered reading *The Red Tent* written by Anita Diamant. I remembered the sense of loss and the emptiness I felt in my life when I had read how women and young girls would gather and bleed together, preparing each other for what was to come, and even those who had long since bled would remain with the younger generations sharing stories and wisdom.

The ache returned but this time it was laced with excitement. This wasn't going to be a depressing time in my life, it was going to be the most liberating time in my life and no matter what life threw at me, I was going to ride the hot, sweaty, chocolate eating moments with grace and gusto! It was time to own my amazing ovaries and just go with the flow... quite literally until it stopped, which according to 'the research' I only had 8 years to go until this 'flow' of the past thirty-three years came to a beautiful hot mess of an end.

The other great thing was I had been a vegetarian on and off all my life so the plant based vegan life has prepared me well. I was a vegetarian most of the time, but when I was pregnant, eating the 'biggest, baddest' rare steak I could find was more desirable than my sexy husband. The more I learnt about industrialised farming the more I was giving up all animal products. I had also given up gluten back in 2010 so I had been ticking all the boxes of preparing my body for menopause without even knowing it... according to my female friends who had turned 'plant based'. Was a plant-based diet the best thing for menopause though? I still didn't know, but like I said before 'poor preparation leads to piss poor performance' and being an over achiever, I now had an even greater desire to ace this menopause business.

With the beginning of my sixth book *Moana*, the first book in *The Sacral Series*, my research took me deeper into the process of womb healing and all things to do with healing after sexual trauma. Some of the research I found said that if there has been sexual trauma then menopause was likely to be worse. Oh great! That's one in three women then that will have a worse menopause because someone violated her.

Sitting on the beach one night after a fire release ritual and sunset swim, I looked out over the Atlantic Ocean and offered gratitude up to the Universe. I was glad I had gone through a deep energy healing and three-hour womb cleansing meditation which had left me exhausted and a sense of relief after literally having given birth to an entity of energy – one which had taken residence inside my body after my own sexual traumas.

Sat there on the beach I thought back to the research and wondered, *How do they know menopause is worse for a woman after sexual trauma? What measure do they have to know how bad the menopause will be if there is sexual trauma?* Looking at the names of all those who had discovered all these 'facts' I noticed a pattern. They were all men.

I then looked through all the research I had been collecting on menopause and sure enough, pretty much all the research out there in the world was written by men. The depressing books were written by men, and the ones which were written by women were so clinical it seemed to me that the women had gone down the clinical route to distance themselves from the reality of what was either to come, or what was actually happening.

Then the thought of gender inequality hit me. Were these women writing the most clinical books out there to prove they could reason and present the data in the most unemotional way possible? To prove they were as worthy of their jobs as scientists to have their research validated in some way. Was I looking for something that wasn't there?

I came to the realisation that it didn't matter why they had written these clinical and depressing books, I needed books about what women experienced, real life experiences of women, ones that didn't depress me to within an inch of my life – and I needed to speak with my older girlfriends about their journeys.

One of my friends told me to keep a great bottle of wine on hand, then remembered I didn't drink. Another told me to make sure I had plenty of KY Jelly with me as it was going to get drier than the Sahara

Desert 'down there'. This I didn't pay much attention to as I was single and celibate so being dryer than the Sahara wasn't going to be an issue, until I met a man worthy of giving up my celibacy – and who knew how long that would take!

The advice of another friend was the was icing on the cake for me because she recommended a vaginal lift! A VAGINAL LIFT? WTAF??? This blew my mind! A vaginal lift? Why? What was going to happen with my vagina? Was it going to end up swinging down by my knees?

I could imagine it, boobs around the waist, vagina on the knees, false teeth in a jar and granny glasses to deal with the apparently soon to be disappearing eyesight, all whilst clutching a bag of knitting, and covered in flour and jam after a Sunday bake off session. Whilst being slightly worried about the female equivalent to brewer's droop, and not a very classy, glamourous or even elegant end to life, I did find this image bloody hilarious!

Having done quite a bit of research by this point the list of symptoms listed out in front of me was growing longer and longer. I started paying attention to the ladies who were now within my personal and professional networks. They made fifty look fabulous, sixty look sexy and seventy look sensual. There was hope at the bottom of the jam jar and I was going to be like these ladies when I grew up and become the wisest witch of all! A burst of excitement hit me and I laughed out loud with the ocean crashing in front of me "Hello Crone Years!! Here I come!"

The walk back along the beach included a sexy confident walk with a wiggle, and the air of confidence I had just gained was wonderful. I knew I would have a few challenges ahead of me, but they now paled into insignificance.

Figuring out how I would know the difference between having hot flushes in the tropics or whether I was just hot would be dealt with as and when it happened. I was now determined to be the smokin' hot sexy Mama kind of hot, even if the hot flushes would make me want to strip off and climb into a deep freeze.

I had also learnt that hot flushes were in fact called hot flashes which then conjured another visual entirely, which I then reframed to the sexy sequin flashes of the sensual art of Burlesque. Yep! I could definitely see me on stage in a pair of fish net tights, hot pants, corset, choker and bowler hat dancing on stage around a chair. On the list of 'Things to achieve' this new vision went – no way was I going to be a grotty grandma!

Since the age of forty I had started to sail around the world so learning that with these hot flashes, also came interrupted sleep patterns. I knew I was going to have to navigate more than just the oceans because when we are crossing oceans or sailing up the coasts doing boat deliveries, we are on a four-hour watch rotation so interrupted sleep patterns are a way of life.

Would these night watches and interrupted sleep patterns be another feather in my cap for acing this menopause journey?

When sailing, my sleep is never deep due to always being in the space between listening for changes in the engine, any tapping noises which shouldn't be happening, as well as listening to the sounds of weather changes, and the delightful sounds of dolphins and whales.

Add into this mix, always listening to the breathing patterns of my two sons as they grew up just in case there was a change in rhythm. Being a writer who wakes up in the middle of the night to write the most amazing ideas and content before falling back to sleep, only to wake up wondering who actually wrote the content because I had no recollection of writing it, my sleep has always been interrupted. This is why I loved Nanna naps in the afternoon... well at any time of the day to be honest (naps are so under rated).

One day as I was crossing the Atlantic on a beautiful three masted barque tall ship, I had just woken up after one of my fabulous naps. Looking out at the horizon a smile rose up from deep within me and I felt a wave of contentment and peace wash over me. In just over a week, I was about to celebrate my forty-second birthday on board this beautiful ship, in the middle of the Southern Atlantic Ocean and although my two sons were not with me in person, this moment was the first moment I felt like my forties were going to be a magical decade for me.

I didn't know how, I didn't know why, but I knew that whatever happened with my body, whether I stayed single for the rest of my days or in a committed loving relationship with a man who had earned the right and proven his worth to be my First Mate, I was going to be just fine. I was in great shape, I ate a plant based non-processed food diet, didn't drink alcohol or smoke any kind of substance, I exercised regularly, and I had a great outlook on life. I was blessed. Really, truly blessed.

Arriving in Las Malvinas, aka The Falkland Islands, I called my two sons and nothing could prepare me for what happened next. My eldest son appeared on the screen with a fully grown goatee and a voice fully broken. Where had my baby gone? And why had no one prepared me for this? I had only been at sea for seven weeks! Was this really how quickly things transformed? This wasn't society or my son telling me he was now a man; this was his own body declaring to the world he was a man. My emotions had gone from a state of bliss to a state of panic and confusion. Did I end my circumnavigation and return back to England so I didn't miss another moment or did I continue to complete this epic world tour researching cultures, women, leadership, parenting and the environment for my Mermaid's Guide series of books?

Before I even had a moment too long to think about it, my son called me out on my thoughts and said "Stop thinking about coming back. You are not happy in the UK; this is not your place anymore. You have to continue this adventure." Tears filled my eyes, and he was right. I wasn't happy in the UK. I had lasted four years in the UK after living out in Egypt and those four years had driven me potty. Now having lived in so many more countries, learning about the world we live in, the human rights abuses, the social injustices, the beauty of the natural world and how various different cultures lived and thrived even with little to no income, and even in the worst conditions imaginable, going back to live in the UK was not an option.

Even being in Las Malvinas made me feel uncomfortable and gave me a deeper dislike for the British Government and military. British Politics had a lot to answer for around the world and I realised I was becoming increasingly disenchanted with all things British. That was until I discovered the thermal underwear, including long johns and thermal long-sleeved vest in *the local store for local people* which were very much needed as the crew and I were heading further south towards Antarctica. I was also probably a tad too excited to see Wilkins Lemon Curd and some good old-fashioned Piccalilli, PG Tips and a plethora of British confectionary which I hadn't seen in years.

Making one last call to my boys before the next few weeks at sea heading into the *'rolling 50s'* in the southernmost part of the Atlantic Ocean, I told them of my great finds and they both started to laugh when I told them about my thermals. "You really are an old lady now mother! Drinking tea, eating piccalilli, followed by lemon curd on toast, all whilst wearing your thermals." Cheeky sods the pair of them, but they were right... I would be drinking tea with piccalilli sandwiches, with lemon curd on toast to follow, whilst wearing my thermals. The only thing they missed off was that I would be reading a book between long periods of time looking out at the ocean watching penguins and dolphins jumping about playing.

The night we left Las Malvinas I couldn't help but smile and giggle away to myself. Bloody thermal underwear! Who would have thought I would be the owner of a pair of thermals at the age of forty-two! So much for being a hot and sexy Mama Burlesquing her way into her fifties! Still, I was warm and cosy, and that was all that mattered.

Those thermals kept me warm all the way up through Southern Chile, Patagonia and Argentina, and it wasn't until I made my way to Brasil that I finally said goodbye to my beloved thermals and embraced my Daisy Duke' denim shorts and bikini tops. Even just changing my wardrobe I felt like I had shed a decade or two off my life, and my mindset. There was something to be said about living in the tropics and being on the beach all day every day, going out diving and snorkelling.

I felt young, I felt as far away from the vision of menopause as possible.

It was during one of my ocean crossing meditations that the idea for this book came floating into my consciousness, and I had to contact the fabulous Clarissa Kristjansson, a woman who had interviewed me for her podcast shortly after I had arrived on land following my three months crossing the Atlantic.

I still didn't know if I had hit the hot and spicy days of perimenopause, but I did know that I was entering the phase of not giving a shit about what others thought about me. The fire and drive within me had taken me and my life to a whole new level of existence. My periods were still visiting every month, naps were still very much a thing but I was going off coffee; and the only time I ever went off coffee was when I was pregnant with my two boys... or rather young men.

Was my dislike of coffee a sign of the menopause? It made sense. Both periods of a woman's life involved huge hormonal changes and as someone who loved coffee, for me to go off coffee was something friends and family found as surprising as me.

It was time for me and Clarissa to have another conversation. I downloaded every episode of her podcast Thriving Thru Menopause. I listened, laughed and lapped up the information and the real-life stories these fabulous women she was interviewing shared with her. My inner witch had been right all along, menopause could be the most empowering time in our life, provided we listened to our bodies. So, I turned up the volume on my soul, my body and I listened.

I felt good. No, I felt great. If I wanted to nap, I napped. If my body didn't want to work out to my Latin Dance Fitness sessions, then I would walk along the beach and go for a swim. If I wanted to go snorkelling or diving I would. The breathing practice, the silence and being in the ocean was my happy place, a place for me to meditate. Surfing had also become a meditation practice for me when I found the right beach. Laying on the board, looking out onto the horizon, finding that spot on the ocean waiting for the right wave to ride... before falling off and being hugged by the ocean ready to go again.

The ocean doesn't care if you are menopausal or not, and this is one of the things I love about her. She is the greatest leveller of life we have, not to mention the entire life source of the planet. Recently as I have embraced what I think are the initial stages of this new empowering stage of my life, I have found myself becoming more ocean. I don't care about the vanity metrics of business, I don't give a rat's arse about the titles people have, nor do I care if people agree with me or not for the way I live my life, I have embodied this new sense of power. This new wave of feminine fire, and when I get my hot flashes, I am reminded I am one hot flash closer to the greatest chapter of my life so far which excites me more than anything, because if I have achieved all I have achieved in life thus far, imagine what is truly possible when I am on the other side of menopause!

There are days when the Mama Fire kicks in and Goddess help anyone who doesn't behave themselves or puts their earphones in when on their phone as three random individuals found out on an overnight coach from Medellin to Santa Marta when I was in Colombia!

There are times when I wake up in the middle of the night thinking about all the things which are weighing heavy on my mind, so I grab my journal and my pen, write down all that is in my mind and then go back to sleep again. If I can't sleep, I just start my day at stupid o'clock and nap later in the day.

I have stopped drinking coffee altogether and now much prefer a green tea over even a black tea. The clarity I have for my business and the legacy I wish to create for the future generations and humanity as a whole has opened up so many more opportunities.

The courage I have to say "No" or simply walk away from situations which no longer feel right, without feeling like I need to explain myself, has increased dramatically.

The confidence to be me, all of me, the giggling, excited, quirky, eccentric, powerful and the brilliant is at an all-time high and I now understand why for years people said "Life begins at forty" because for me it has with the awakening of the menopause.

As women we have been led to believe our life is over when we hit the menopause, but for me life is only just beginning. I have had thirty years of bleeding for a week every month, and I have survived and thrived every month. I have given birth to my two sons, my businesses, to community regeneration projects, written more than a dozen books, lived and worked in over fifty countries, survived and thrived sexual traumas, the Egyptian Uprising and the Plandemic, learnt and achieved so much more than I ever dreamed possible.

And if I can achieve all I have achieved in the first forty years of my life without the powerful awakening within me the menopause is bringing, then all I can say is "Buckle up Batesy! This is going to be one hell of an adventure!"

Reflections

Reflections

Reflections

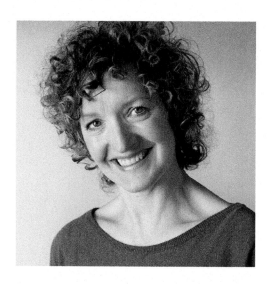

FIONA WHITFIELD
UK

Freedom from Die-t Facilitator, guiding women to build a strong foundation.

Let's look at the word diet. Dieting is not what people think it is. There is a clue in the word diet isn't there?! Die – t.

It's not about you getting thinner and fitter, it's about control. Control of your energy, your body, your finances, your sovereignty, your muchness. It's patriarchal bullshit. Women diet because they don't have power over who they are. And this is where Fiona comes in. She is here to facilitate your growth of all things beyond the Die-t. To stop control of food and exercise, of your size, what you say, and think and do. To stop allowing coercion or gaslighting. To regain your sovereignty in all its glory. She collaborates *with* you so you can allow your muchness, your 'enough-ness,' to come shining through. To let go of labels such as needy, too much, too intense, not enough, too sensitive, moody, autistic, HSP, whatever labels you've been given and to know that it is more than ok to be totally and unapologetically you.

To connect with Fiona visit https://thelifereboot.co.uk

Chapter Three

FUCK IT IN YOUR FIFTIES!

I was a forty-two-year-old fitness coach, training to be a nutritional therapist, when a sentence really jumped out at me during one of the lectures. Being a bit slow to process things, I was always behind as I tried to make sense of things in my note taking, when the clouds parted (metaphorically) and I heard "How a woman manages her menopause is directly linked to the number of stressors in her life. The body will prioritise stress hormones over the sex hormones, so if she is experiencing high stress, this will impact her experience of the menopause"

Shit. I was pretty fucked then!

Unexpectedly, my brother had died a few months prior to me starting my three year training. I had gone through two miscarriages in the last couple of years with another one to shortly follow.

I couldn't see how I could destress those events from my life.

I also had a five-year-old son who had just started in reception class that year and my husband was a workaholic Disney Dad. We had a nice house and '*fancy shmancy*' holidays, but he was out the house for long hours and often away in the week. I felt like a single mum in the week. Thankfully, he was at home at weekends to do the fun stuff with our son while I was at college.

Life felt a long way from stress free.

What the fuck was I doing?

As a classic children's nursery rhyme sung by Michael Rosen says, "We're going on a bear hunt, it's going to be a big one .... you can't go over it, you can't go round it, you have to go through it".

I stumbled along as best I could. Trying to apply some of the things I was learning at college. Eating as well as I could, going to the gym to burn off the stress of feeling guilty for letting my son have pesto pasta or fish fingers every night of the week, guilty for not sprouting my own seeds and guilty for not knitting my own underwear. I still managed to be at the school gate every morning and after school, arranging play dates for my boy and meeting other mums, trying to have my own social life. And somehow fitting in as much studying as my frazzled brain could take. I had barely grieved for my brother or the babies who were not born, I was way too busy white-knuckling my way through life.

I was saying yes to stuff, to nights out, charity work, present buying, cake making, art therapy, because that's what you do, right? I seemed to be doing what everyone around me was doing. Like I was on some kind of weird conveyor belt, going through the motions of life. Inside my head I was screaming, and occasionally sobbing out loud.

I had no clue this was all conditioning. I was living a life that other people had told me was the right way to live.

I was a right mess. Emotions all over the place, sweating in bed, flinging the covers off, on, off, on. Feeling like I wanted to stab my husband if he even so much as thought "old menopausal bag". Angry one minute, sobbing the next. I can't even remember if I was too stubborn to ask for help or too bloody unaware that I was in need of it.

I remember a cake throwing session with a friend one evening. Our boys were at karate together and both of us were on the verge of tears. We had gone up onto the Downs and decided throwing was better than eating. There was lots of shouting and swearing about our partners – it was a very therapeutic night and it gave me an inkling that there was another way through this. Though it did feel a bit of a waste of bloody good cake. At least the sheep would have benefitted.

I ended up at the doctor to say I was struggling to cope; my emotions were all over the place. She somewhat unsympathetically wanted to prescribe me anti-depressants. I declined. I didn't have a mental health issue! (So, I thought) I just wanted someone to listen to me and agree it was shit, I wanted a good night's sleep. I wanted someone to understand. I didn't want anti-fucking-depressants!!!

So, what do you do when the medical options available to you are not acceptable to you? I looked elsewhere. I was determined to find a way to help myself. I attended a training course to help women at 'the menopause stage', (may as well help others too, right?) and taking the attention off me was a good distraction and helped numb all the mood swings and the crazy thoughts.

The training helped me cope and I also helped others along the way with Menopause Workshops. Nutrition. Fitness. Self-Care.

I learnt a lot of the theory, thinking that was what was missing.

The actual menopause is your last period. It's almost like the full stop at the end of a sentence. It's the peri and pre menopause (the lead up to the cessation of your menstruation) which can be the hot flushing, high intensity time. The time when you're likely to be the butt of the menopause 'jokes', and the time you're most likely to give someone a good slug round the ear, right? Or a right verbal telling off.

I remember being aware that something was changing, shortly after a volcano of rage and frustration building in my body led to a feisty rant at my husband about the state of our marriage. Normally I would have been a right people pleaser or biting my lip, and having a whinge afterwards, rather than rocking the boat. But I had got to the stage where I could say what was welling up. It was yelling inside of me to be spoken.

As the words came out of my mouth, it was like my head had lifted up enough to peer out over the parapet and I began to actually start to see what the hell was going on. Was this really my life? How the hell did I get here? What on earth was I doing?

I wish I could say it was a real "Ta Dah!" moment when everything in my life began to change. It was more a mini ta-dah, followed by a slow drip feed. An anti-climax of epic proportions. The dots had started to join, but in small clusters. This was the genius of menopause starting to peek through…. I was starting my real caterpillar into a butterfly metamorphosis, but it was rather longer than I would have liked.

From my menopause training, I knew that oestrogen had over four hundred functions in the body. In the menopause workshops I ran, I was sharing with women what the best foods for hormonal balance were, how to exercise to maintain muscle mass and bone strength. How best to sit on the loo to use your pelvic floor muscles correctly (a pile of books under your feet or a squatty potty, in case you didn't know!). How to 'do' self-care. Giving women space to ask questions, and all was good, but everyone was way too polite to be say what they really wanted or to throw themselves on the floor in an emotional puddle. It would have been amazing if they had!

What I didn't truly get, until it happened, was that as your levels of oestrogen fall, your desire to nurture and care for others also declines. And as oestrogen falls, the relative level of testosterone rises to also help you to be that little bit more self-centred. It's like the veil of oestrogen starts to slowly fall away from your body and you feel like the real you can emerge out into the world.

For someone who was a near lifelong people pleaser, this declining oestrogen was going to massively impact my life in ways I hadn't a clue about at the time. I thought it would be a matter of white knuckling through the hot sweats, bitchy mood swings, low libido, dry vagina, emotional wreckage that was perimenopause, then sit back as life got back to normal.

WRONG!!

What NO-ONE ever tells you is that you may feel your old life fall away as and when you no longer tolerate how things used to be, particularly if you were used to doing things for others and not honouring yourself along the way.

PEOPLE PLEASING AND PERFECTIONISM INTERVAL

Let me interrupt the story to talk about people pleasing and perfectionism. I don't think you can get to the epiphany of menopause, to truly appreciate the gift of it, if you haven't first been a people pleaser and/or perfectionist.

Let me explain.

Many women, growing up in the UK in the sixties or seventies in particular, were brought up in a patriarchal culture, the men went out to work and the women were still (by and large) the ones to stay at home and raise the kids. This was the norm for me and for most of my friends when I was a teenager. The men were mainly the ones who had the power and the women were the ones to obey. Girls were encouraged to be 'good' and 'nice'. By 'good' I mean quiet and subservient *shudders* and 'nice' which was all about being pleasant and polite, not upsetting or offending someone. Being AGREEABLE. I used to get particularly pissed off that these 'nice' and 'good' labels weren't being extended to my brother, who was annoyingly naturally studious and quiet. I remember my mum telling me to just agree with my dad, rather than argue the toss

This makes my hackles rise up even now! I see how I was literally taught to put others' (especially men's) needs before my own, and how this conditioning influenced the first forty-nine years of my life including two marriages. It's a huge relief that I made it to my fifties and I can finally identify and honour my own needs!

Some signs to know if you're a people pleaser:
- You don't realise you have your own needs
- You generally say yes when people ask you a favour
- You say 'no' when you mean 'yes' and 'yes' when you mean 'no'
- You feel guilty for saying no
- You feel resentful when you do something for someone else
- You're known as the 'helpful one' who everyone turns too
- You don't feel able to speak up and say what you think
- You say "Sorry!". A lot.

People pleasing is pretty disempowering but identifying it is the first step to overcoming it, and the same goes for the ugly sister of people pleasing - perfectionism.

And before you start thinking "Hang on a minute, I'm not a perfectionist!" let me explain my version of the term. People used to tell me I was a perfectionist and I NEVER got it. As far as I was concerned, I was far from a perfectionist. I'm not particularly good at anything and I mistakenly thought that being a perfectionist was being someone who wanted to be good at something and kept practicing over and over again, trying really hard to be better at it. As it turns out this isn't always correct. If you're the kind of person who does something and is dissatisfied and repeats it once or even more, and you do that with any kind of regularity, then you have perfectionist tendencies. It's the dissatisfaction with what you have done, whether it's painting, baking, running, present wrapping, posting on social media or putting on your eyeliner. It may just be your own judgement of not being good enough, but it could also be that you fear being judged by others. Being cast out of the tribe, so to speak. The ultimate fear for some.

Both people pleasing and perfectionism appear to have something in common at their root and that's the inability to be truly you. To be accepted for who you are, to be loved exactly as you are, warts and all. And I think we all fucking deserve that.

Here's my two penn'orth to help overcome PP and P:

- Practise having boundaries. And if that feels too difficult start by saying 'NO' when someone asks you to do something you don't want to and 'YES' when you're asked to do something you DO want to
- Practise being good enough, aka imperfect. Oh my God, the joy of this!!! I can't tell you how liberating it is! Next time you do something you would normally have two or more goes at before you 'get it right', try doing it once and then, LEAVE IT! Honestly, it's brilliant.
- If all else fails. Become menopausal.

BACK TO THE STORY....

Apart from my rebellious teenage years, which my mum still delights in the fact she knew all the 'weirdo people' in my home town because they were friends of mine (I bloody loved those creative, outside-the-box thinking people), I had definitely fallen into the trap of being a people pleaser, acting nice, trying to be 'good', to not eat too much, to keep quiet, not to rock the boat and basically I learnt to pretend things were ok, even if they weren't. Especially if they weren't!

This was all in an attempt to fit in, to be accepted, to be liked (the ultimate end game for a people pleaser). I didn't know any better, I wasn't aware of anyone who was doing it differently. Like so many other women, I was just stuck on the conveyor belt of life, not questioning, just doing.

After nearly five decades, it was all about to unravel.......

I was forty-nine and could feel inklings of my teenage self, starting to stir. This feistiness was rising and I couldn't push it down even if I wanted to.

It wasn't just that I started swearing more. I was dissatisfied. With my life but more importantly with *me!* How could I be happy in my marriage, if I wasn't happy in myself?

With that new realisation, it was time to address the problem.

I checked for holes in my fitness and self-care. I doubled down on my 'clean eating', did more exercise, booked in hot stone massages and spa days with my friends. Had some weekends away and date nights with the hubs in an attempt to rekindle our marriage.

I even addressed some of the things that were nagging at me. At fifty, I got that tattoo I'd always wanted to get but thought I 'shouldn't'. I had a dramatic haircut and let my grey shine through, despite comments from various people telling me I'd look 'old' (you mean my age?!) Who gives a fuck what anyone else thinks?!

All that made me feel slightly better but I was still annoyingly dissatisfied. Was this it? Is this life I had the one I had to put up with? It's how I like to think Columbus came to discover America? He was just plain dissatisfied with life in Italy and all that fucking pasta.

Then quite by chance, I eventually 'came across' the docufilm Embrace.

After watching it, I realised something had clicked. It spoke to me loud and clear with the "embrace your body exactly as it is" message and how pervasive diet culture and the media campaigns surrounding it is. The subliminal messages are everywhere. My eyes now wide open, I realised that I had bought into this messaging, hook, line and sinker. It was clear to me that dieting, 'clean eating', exercise your way to a 'perfect' body programmes I had done for decades were NOT the answer to my dissatisfaction with myself. It was the media messaging telling me that I needed to be thinner, in order to be happier. It was such a relief to finally see what a load of bollocks that truly is.

DIET CULTURE AND MENOPAUSE

Being a serial dieter for (coughs) thirty something years, AND being in the field of health and wellbeing, it came as a huge surprise when I started to see the diet industry with fresh eyes for what it really is.

A multi-billion-dollar agency that for the most part has ZERO interest in your health and wellbeing, but instead one that relies on the FAILURE of its own systems to keep you in its clutches.

I know!! Shocking, isn't it?

If you've been on diets in some way shape or size for some time, menopause could be the time to get clarity around diet culture. Maybe you've used exercise or 'clean eating' in order to control your size or shape? I call this dieter mentality if the end goal is to be THINNER or SMALLER than you currently are. Once you get the idea of how it's all a big con, it is really hard to get back on the diet/exercise bandwagon. You will have too much relative testosterone to be part of it anymore and won't want to be part of a system that is corrupt and fucked up!

BUT…. it's equally liberating and terrifying to stop dieting if that's all you've known.

Liberating to know that you are taking matters into your own hands, that you are old enough and resourceful enough to do this on your own.

Think of all you have achieved in your life! Of course, you can be ok without feeding into big diet!! Go you!

And terrifying because you've relied on dieting SO much over the years. Relied on the quick fix to lose those few pounds for that thing you wanted to look good for, having bust a gut and sweated in out in the gym or at bootcamp three times a week to tone your thighs and bum. What do you do when left to your own devices?? What if you turn into a sofa slob?!!

So, here's the thing. Diets don't work. long term. It's like taking pain killers for a headache you have constantly, rather than sort out the cause of the headache (Bad eyesight? Poor lighting? Neck misalignment? Dehydrated? Toxin overload? etc.)

If you still aren't convinced it's time to stop dieting, do a little digging into diet culture and patriarchy. There's enough info there to keep you entertained for a few hours – months even! It should have you ditching the monthly slimming club subs quicker than prepping a slim-a-shake. And if you want something to get you a little more riled up – check out dieting and racism… Don't say I didn't warn you!

Menopause means you are no longer content with slapping a band aid on things. You can no longer put up with things that don't sit right with you. You want, no NEED, to do it differently. What do you do instead of relying on counting calories, points, macros and the like?

You learn to trust. You learn the subtle messages your body is giving you about what you want and when you want it. And you do it by listening in and honouring your body. Don't expect to be able to do it all, to learn the method in a week or a month or even a year because there's no 'quick fix' here - why did we ever think there would be? But you're now in it for the long game. You're now in it so that for the remaining thirty or so years of your life, you can do all the things you want, with all the people you want to do it with. Yes?

If that all feels too big, stressful and scary, you find some support.

Find your own champion who can help you when things get sticky or some fellow newbie diet rebels to do it with.

As Dr Sara Gottfried (2021) says on her Facebook site, "Women have a biological imperative to tend and befriend when under stress". We tend to do better when we are around other women.

There are lots of people teaching intuitive eating, body confidence and, as I do, learning to honour your body.

Here are my top tips to listening to your own body and what she wants:

- Surfing the Urge: This one is GREAT if you are a snacker or an emotional eater. It works best if it's a snack actually, but any food will do. You get your food, let's say a biscuit and a cuppa and right as you lift the biscuit to your mouth, you pause. Literally. And do you notice why you're eating? What is going through your mind? Your body? What potentially jumbled weird messaging is your body telling you about why you should consume that biscuit. No judgements here, (nice try) just notice! Journal or make note of what comes up for you. This is so useful to be able to understand your triggers for eating, your reasons. And of course, you then get to eat the biscuit. If you still want to.

- Be More French: Another awareness exercise (can you see the theme?). Particularly good if you eat mindlessly or quickly. Choose a meal when you can create a bit of time. Prepare something you really enjoy, this one is better if it's a meal, as if you are going on a date (which is true, but it's with yourself). Set the table, maybe with a tablecloth, put a candle on, some flowers in a vase, or both. Maybe even dress up (or down! Your preference) and S-L-O-W everything down. Take a moment to appreciate the meal before you start eating, by looking at the colours and the textures and the smell of your food. Maybe even think with a French accent?! "Zis food, eet smells marvel-yurr" (Too much?!) When you eat, take a bite at a time, with sassy Frenchness and put your fork down in between bites. Taste. Savour. Enjoy. If you really were French, you would be smoking a Gauloise by now and be supping some rich French wine, this is optional. (Apologies to my French friends, none of whom eat this way, but please don't spoil my romantic imaginings of French people in days gone by)

- Let Your Body Move & Groove – forget what all the flipping guru's say about what exercise you SHOULD do and find what it is your body WANTS to do. One thing's for sure, if you don't love what you do (or if it doesn't love you back), then you won't keep it up, even if it's the most 'perfect' thing for you to do. What did you love to do when you were little? How would you finish this sentence – "I've always wanted to try xxx?" Is it archery? Walking football? Rowing? Synchronised swimming? Dragon boat racing? Wheelchair basketball? Tai Chi? Chair burlesque?! There really is something for everyone and I love when people find their thing! Be creative and see where it goes…. And before you start thinking you're too old for blah, I recently started a pole dancing class (age fifty-seven) run by a bloody fabulous woman in her sixties!!

The funny thing is, that once you decide to stop dieting or following someone else's rules about being healthy, when all food and movement is on the menu for you to choose from, so to speak, you may decide that you actually don't like the things you thought you should be eating/doing. Giving yourself permission to be the person who chooses what is right for you, is really powerful. And learning to have fun and enjoy the experiment of finding this out too.

There is also a strong chance you find a liberating acceptance about your shape and size and end up feeling that you don't give a shit if people don't like how you look. Especially once the people pleasing genes disappear! It is no-one else's fucking business what you look like. So sod 'em! (as we say in England!)

Okay, so if dieting wasn't the answer, what was?

Time To Investigate More.

I started to interrogate me a little more. What did I want to do? What was I all about? What was I doing for other people instead of doing for me?

At the time I had a good friend who was good at putting herself first. My then husband commented on how selfish she was when she went off on a singing holiday to Spain. Odd because I thought how similar they were! He had gone off on a fishing holiday to the US, and on a skiing holiday by himself, but he didn't see the similarities in that at all.

Rather than thinking if her husband didn't like her taking time for herself, that was their business, nothing to do with anyone else, I was really envious of her for doing her own thing. Not many other women I knew would do that. I had grown up in a world where men wouldn't think twice about going off and doing their thing, but when it comes to their female counterpart, that's a different matter. I came up with loads of excuses why I wouldn't do that which were all connected to me being 'needed' to look after my kid, my dog, the house, my work, blah blah blah. But I didn't have the balls, or the 'vadge[1]' enough to do it myself.

What did my friend have that I didn't? How could I do something like that? What was stopping me? Why had I never noticed this before?! It had taken menopause for the dissatisfaction in my life to become clear.

I did what many people surely do in that position and fell head long into self-development. When you no longer have 'Big Diet' to occupy your time and energy, you find somewhere else to look and that's inside.

Self-development. Self-help. Personal development. Self-improvement. Call it what you like. I don't particularly relate to any of those terms. I feel it's a 'Learning to Be Yourself'.

One of the first things that smacked me round the face quite early on (and it was and still is a work in progress) was all the things we do because we think we should. So much conditioning, living by other people's rules, but not questioning.

I noticed how much I used to bitch and moan about doing things, but not ever doing anything different.

Do said thing.

Moan about doing it.

Do said thing again.

---

1   Slang term for vagina in England

Moan about doing it.

And I was moaning about other people who used to bitch and moan too! I couldn't see that I was holding up a mirror to myself. Yet.

But as I started to become more aware, I noticed how much of my life was about what I thought I wanted to do, with very little idea what I actually did want. I was so conditioned, I never thought to question what I really wanted. I didn't even realise I had needs, let alone thinking about getting them met. No wonder I was envious of my friend speaking up and doing something she wanted to do. I now find it incredible (without judgement) that I had got to fifty something and to have been so unconscious!

I felt like the more aware I was becoming, the less of a clue I had of WHAT to do.

But I needed to do something. Anything was better than sitting still and not attempting to improve my life. It wasn't going to improve by itself.

I began trying different things. I read books and became a bit of a e-programme junkie. I started making minor changes. Like delegating some of things I didn't like (cleaning) or ditching them completely (ironing). If anyone wanted their work/school shirts ironing, they could damn well do their own.

I found ways to make some of the more humdrum things more enjoyable – like meeting a friend to walk our dogs – for me dog walking is great but only when I don't have to do it EVERY day.

Walking dog on own every day = pissed off, irritable and total victim = not good.

Walking with friend = social plus exercise = good.

These small but significant changes were having an effect, but I was still avoiding the elephant in the room. I was trying to change external factors in order to feel better in myself. I had no idea that was the case at the time. Hindsight is marvellous, isn't it?!

It's like having a cake that isn't great but spending your time trying to make the icing ok and the top of it look like a pro had worked their magic.

None of my friends seemed to notice. No one pointed out that I was acting strangely. I felt strange, but they didn't seem to notice. Was I hiding it that well? Were they busy going through their own shit? In retrospect I realise I had gotten so used to pretending and convincing myself all was ok, that I was convincing others too. I was settling for a less than life and not saying anything, keeping it all in. Until I couldn't.

Now that I live in a world where proper interactive communication is the norm rather than the exception, I wonder why I never questioned the superficial conversations I had been having for all of my life?

If, in our early years no one has modelled how to communicate effectively, how to have difficult conversations, how to deal with emotions in a healthy way, then we can all to easily find ways to distract and suppress our emotions or use different strategies, like crying or shouting, in order to be heard. It shows how what we learn as little sponges, in the first seven years, has such an effect on our lives. How we can accept these behaviours as normal and keep choosing partners and relationships where we are repeating these patterns of behaviour. So many opportunities to learn!

I was great at practicing pretence, pre menopause. Queen of the F word. "Oh, I'm fine", even if I felt far from it. I had learnt to be 'happy' at all costs.

Happy = good. All other emotions = bad.

Do you remember 'Fake it till you make it'? I wondered why I had a strong aversion to that phrase!

Where Did This All Come From?

Being raised by parents who had been through the war meant that they were not in touch with their emotions. They had to internalise a lot and not show their emotions, when they were growing up. They learned to try and hold it together as a way of getting through that horrendously scary time.

My parents adopted a dear little boy in the early 1960's. He was agreeable and polite and was able to entertain himself with toy trains and books. A 'good' boy. So, they were in for a shock when three years later they got pregnant and along came me, a lively, curious, playful child, with a whole bag full of emotions to express. They had no idea what to do when I started to use them! It felt like they would do what they could to stop them from escaping from me. My dad would hold up the paper and 'hide' behind it when I was being emotional, and my mum would tell me I was too intense and ask why I couldn't be more like my brother. I learnt to find ways to cope, and food became a great self-soother for when unhappiness, discomfort, anger, irritation etc. came up. There was no safe space for emotions with parents who had shut down their own during WWII.

The only acceptable way of being, was to be 'happy', and whatever you do, don't get into anything too deep. Keep it light, keep it superficial and above all, PRETEND you are ok! And of course, 'good girls' didn't show their emotions, it wasn't fucking ladylike!

Not for the first time did I question if I was adopted. Surely, I was in the wrong family? I didn't feel like I fit in in the slightest.

I became bulimic, squashing down those emotions with food and then vomiting them back up with guilt of eating. Oh shit! I'm supposed to be 'good' and 'good' is thin - not stuffing down five cream cakes within the space five minutes.

These squashed emotions were somehow locked in my body until …. can I have a drum roll please??? The great menopause unveiling! It's like someone unlocked them from prison and they all rushed up to be heard and wouldn't shut up.

At first, I was totally overwhelmed by all this intensity of feeling. I wasn't used to it; I didn't recognise this weirdness and the only option seemed to let 'them' out to run riot. It helped to sweat it out in the gym if I was angry or cry it out if I was sad. Going for a drive to sing and shout worked at times but after being 'let out' my emotions would crop up at the most inconvenient times and it wasn't always appropriate to rage it out. It was a bit like teenage boys getting erections at inappropriate moments! There were mutterings about me being 'menopausal' and then the eye rolling and jokes about hot flushes would follow.

And glad as I was that I was allowing myself to feel emotions, I still tried to 'get them out the way' as soon as possible. Especially anger.

Cake throwing was an expensive waste of good cake.

So, I was bloody delighted to train in energy therapy and learn about the frequency of emotions and getting another lightbulb moment around learning "Emotions are for feeling!" To understand that they actually have a purpose, we can learn from them, then we can move on. We don't have to be hostages to our emotions. E- motions are literally energy in motion, originating from the Latin word meaning to agitate or to move out. Each emotion has a different energetic frequency and we can shift our emotions with our thoughts and our movements.

For someone who was emotionally barren for fifty years, learning that emotions had a purpose, that they were valid, was like manna from heaven.

Apparently the basic emotions of joy, anger, sadness, fear, love, like, dislike, were first identified in first century China and that these 'primitive' emotions are hard wired in us, meaning they are quick to appear as they have a survival element to them.

If we have emotional shame from our formative years and then add to that the menopausal rollercoaster of changing hormones, it's no wonder some of us women feel completely emotionally overwhelmed at times – especially when no one talks about this aspect.

How to practice emotional wellness

- Find your buddies. Get together with other women going through something similar (social media, especially Facebook, is often handy for finding a support group). Choose the right size group for you whether it's a couple of local women or a large, organised group online – they are out there, and they can help. Make sure you feel safe to speak your truth and that there is no judgement (otherwise wrong group). Remember, women tend to do better with other women in times of stress and it can feel good to let it all out and know there are others feeling the same. It might be useful to be with women who are slightly older than you and have experienced what you're going through. Don't hang out with people who say, "Oh my menopause was a breeze and just sailed through it". Not helpful and far too smug!

- Journal your feelings as they come up, talk to a (willing) friend, or move your body – walk, dance, run, swim. Whatever helps you process your emotions easiest. Movement helps to shift emotions, 'up the scale' (to higher frequency emotions, starting with contentment and moving toward love, joy or peace) and it helps to learn good body awareness.
- Find ways to diffuse/offset stress. Menopausal women often get more stress reactive, so we activate the stress hormones more easily and quickly (yeah, it's a bummer but it means we should really listen to this and down tools a bit/a lot). Actually, it's imperative that if you can't ditch your job and go and live on a desert island by yourself for a few years, that you find ways to do something. It's worth a conversation with your nearest and dearest to explain it's a biological necessity and for their safety (*wink*) to slow down for a few years.
  o What exactly CAN you do?
  o What do you love doing?
  o What do you need more/less of in your life? A little something regularly is better than going all out and not being able to keep things up.
  o Do you need more peace and tranquillity?
  o More nourishment, spiritual or physical?

And I can pretty much guarantee you need to laugh more. Laughter is great at diffusing the sympathetic nervous system (stress hormones), boosts your endorphins (feel good hormones) plus it improves your immunity and a host of other health benefits. And it's pretty much at our fingertips – at the click of a mouse to find some comedy gold on the old internet.

This was NOT something I managed to do well at all. To be honest, I was pretty shit at it. I learnt it all in dribs and drabs (where was THIS book when I needed it?!) over quite a few years.

I slowly learnt, sorry s - l - o - w - l - y learnt, that proper radical self-care is the antidote to stress. I knew it, but had to experience it in my body, to embody it, before I GOT it.

I think anytime we go through a big life event, it's time to properly look after ourselves, tune in to our own needs and screw what everyone else says. Or maybe it hits home more to say if you want to continue to feel discontent with your life, then continue the people pleasing, the giving your power away to another diet/exercise/self-development program where you are not cultivating awareness of how YOUR body is responding, what YOUR body truly wants. Ouch?

Menopause and its tricky hormonal shenanigans may just be the springboard you need for a life reboot of sorts (warning, you may end up living a truly authentic life!).

Women at menopause have on average another thirty years to live. That's a lot of time to be living a dissatisfied, disempowered, less than life, isn't it?

Radical self-care and all the selves (self-love, self-compassion, self-awareness, self-kindness, self-respect) is proper. It's not the 'pretty, Insta type selfie-care", it's the cry-til-you're-a-snotty-mess, try, fail, try, fail again, try something different, succeed, rinse and repeat version. Not for the faint hearted. But the rewards can be beautiful. Though you will need to choose your team wisely, a support network is pretty vital - it's bloody hard to go it alone.

I know I bang on about self-care quite a lot, and I get that you probably know quite a bit already, so I've devised a little quiz of sorts to 'test' your Self Care Knowledge. Are you ready?

Which of the following can be considered self-care (and extra points if you can identify those which are radical self-care)? And can you spot any red herrings?

- Eating food which is nutritious and good for you
- Eating cake (maybe home-made chocolate cake?)
- Exercising doing something you love
- Exercising when you're tired
- Doing exercise because a fitness coach said you should do it
- Having a nap at 11 am
- Going to bed early instead of going out with friends
- Going out with friends instead of going to bed early!

- Saying No to something you want to do
- Saying Yes to something someone else wants you to do
- Expressing your anger
- Not expressing your sadness

I wonder, did you want to look ahead to see what the answers were?! I always used to do that with magazine quizzes, so I could 'fix' the answers in order to feel better about myself – I definitely didn't feel good enough back then.

The truth is there are only three red herrings. (Oops sorry I lied about extra points!) All the other answers could be classed as self-care and even radical self-care *IF* they are things which feel good and nourishing and what you need to be doing AT THAT TIME and *IF* you don't feel pressurised or coerced into doing something.

Do you have that well-meaning friend who tells you "C'mon, let's go out to the pub, you'll feel better if you do!" when you've just explained you are dog tired and, on the floor, exhausted? Hence why the going out instead of going to bed early IS self-care, if your heart is telling you to go, rather than your pushy mate!

Even the red herrings could possibly be self-care under certain circumstances.

Doing exercise, a fitness coach said you 'should' do – this might be something you've said you are a little cautious about and as a result they may be encouraging you to try in a positive and supportive way = self-care. Some buff trainer yelling at you to do "ten more press ups!!! Let's go!!!" is only self-care if you manage to punch them on the nose!

Similarly, with saying yes to something someone else wants you to do and not expressing your sadness. There could be circumstances where both of these might be self-care. I'll let your imagination come up with some creative suggestions for these!

Obviously, there are many more things under the self-care umbrella – your thoughts and beliefs, your actions, who you hang around, what you say and do, what you consume, as well as what you eat and how you move, can all affect your energy and how you feel. All these things are connected, they all form part of your self-care. The radical part comes in when you realise that it is non-negotiable to make choices which support your wellbeing. That you are the one to have the control over decisions around your self-care. What you read/watch on tv – does it inform you and make you feel empowered or make you feel angry/anxious? Who do you spend most of your time with – how do you feel when you are with those people?

I was completely clueless about all this at my menopause, but with the awareness that everything impacts you on a physical, emotional, mental, energetic or spiritual level, you are empowered to decide whether something you are doing is working for you or not. It's almost like you are running the company (the company being your body) and you are also the CEO of that company. You alone get to decide what your needs are, how you want to live your life - what's working, what isn't.

Start with something simple - what things are non-negotiable for your everyday well-being? Choose two to five and do them daily.

I call this your essential well-being kit, and only you will know what that is. It could be to prioritise sleep, or to have a great breakfast. To journal or meditate every morning. Or lie in bed. Drink two litres of water. Meet a friend. Have sex. Have chocolate. You get the idea – don't overthink it!

And finally, can we talk about joy?? Too many women I talk to around menopause seem to have lost the capacity for boundless joy. The dictionary definition of joy is *"the emotion evoked by well-being, success, or good fortune or by the prospect of possessing what one desires"*

I experience it as feeling a sort of intense pleasure in seeing or hearing something or being with someone which makes you feel so present and connected and fully open hearted. I often feel lost trying to find words, as if they are inadequate to explain something. To me joy can be 'quiet' or 'loud' but it is definitely the icing on the cake in life. To have moments of joy are what make life special. Watching that sunrise, seeing those magnificent views, hearing that music, sharing laughter with friends, moving your body in a way that feels so good, experiencing xxxxx (fill in the blank) for the first time.

If you are menopausal and living a life less than, then joy is your North Star. Find the things you absolutely love to do and do them. All the time. And when you do that and you come alive... THIS is true radical self-loving-care.

It truly breaks my heart when I see women giving their power away – when we have the capacity to be so blooming powerful! In both the fierce Mama Bear (and you don't have to have had children to have this) and the gentle caring way.

Conditioning and culture have much to answer for disempowering women. As of 2021, women in Saudi Arabia still don't have the vote. That blows my mind. And makes me more determined to be my own advocate, to feel fully empowered to make my own decisions about my life and my body, to be able to speak and be heard. To be imperfectly perfect trying to live as authentically as I can and to help other women on the road to that too.

I hope you feel inspired to do the same for yourself. Find your buddies, your support team and get started on some rip roaring, toe curling, radical, joyful self-loving care!

Reflections

Reflections

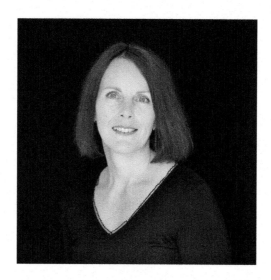

SU WINSBURY
UK

Spiritual Mentor, Empowerment Coach & Energy Alchemist to Conscious Change-Makers, Rebels and Leaders of the New Paradigm

Su is a truth seeker, visionary and champion of change-makers mastering their innate energy so they create powerful impact and transformation in the world.

With a no-fluff attitude towards personal development and spiritual growth, she will take you on a tour of your inner world, unseen shadows and deepest subconscious so that you connect with your true potential and create in complete energetic alignment with your soul.

Su blends deep, powerful energy practices and intuition with more than twenty years' experience in entrepreneurship, wellbeing and healing to empower you to own your truth with authority and influence.

www.suwinsbury.com

Chapter Four

MENOPAUSE: BRINGING HOME THE BODY, MIND, AND SOUL

We often forget that we are so much more than a body.

We are given this physical home to inhabit, to grow, learn and evolve. It is the most incredible and intricately designed piece of creation – as is everything in nature – which we are gifted as humans yet so often we fail to truly appreciate, respect, or honour this vessel.

We are quick to curse it when it doesn't serve us well, has a bit of blip in the system or brings us difficult changes of life but we rarely remember to thank it when it is working beautifully. We take it for granted, use it and abuse it.

From my teens I knew that there was something way more to us than just the body and the mind. I didn't know what that greater part was but became fascinated by the concepts of the soul and spirit. Unfortunately, back in the bygone days of the early eighties, we didn't have the wonders of a quick search at the touch of a button, we only had the local library filled with the delights of proper books, an appreciation of which has never left me. There is nothing quite like the satisfaction of turning the pages, popping in your bookmark (or dare I say with advance apologies to our lovely publisher, turning the corner of the page over) and feeling the physical presence of the words in your hands.

Anyway, after reading copious stories of the afterlife by Doris Stokes [1] as that was all I could find in my village library, my research came to a standstill. Gin, New Romantics, big hair and boys came into my life and filled the void for many years until a random advertisement in the local newspaper popped into view offering an introduction to spiritual healing.

At that moment, I came home to a lost part of me. Learning to connect with energy and healing was like putting the most comfortable cosy pair of slippers on after wearing badly fitting shoes for years.

It was easy, it felt so natural and it ignited some very old wisdom from deep inside my soul.

So, what does all this have to do with menopause?

Nothing, and yet everything.

Menopause is a rite of passage, an evolution not just of the body but of the mind and soul as we move through this human experience of a life. It isn't just an inconvenient, often nightmarish experience that only the female of the species at best endures, at worst suffers. It is the third major transition in the feminine form, the move into the wise, intuitive and potent woman that has often been waiting to burst forth into reality.

I want to take you on a journey of delving into the body, mind and the soul through menopause. Having spent years working with energy, health and wellbeing, I have deep insight into the workings of the body and how we can support it more powerfully on every level. I also offer my theory on how we can help ourselves and other women move through this phase with more ease, fewer symptoms and more love for who we are.

This is dedicated to my dear friend Louise who departed this earth very suddenly during the writing process. Thank you for the good times and the love my friend.

---

1   Doris Stokes 1920-1987, was a British spiritualist, self-proclaimed medium and author.

LET'S GET PHYSICAL

"It must be my coil running out. It's been there nearly five years, so it must be that - it's at the end of its life. I need to get it changed. Or just give my body a break."

That was how I viewed the increase in heat I was experiencing during the night. Waves of intense heat, not every night but certainly becoming noticeable. For someone who feels the cold, the sudden bursts of night time glow were obvious.

I was forty-one, my marriage was finally hitting breaking point after several years of sticking it together with plasters, tape and a huge dollop of denial and my two young boys were about to get a huge shock as their family disintegrated. The Universe conspired to throw in a couple of other biggies for good measure as it likes to work in threes − my cousin lost her argument with cancer and my mum was diagnosed with breast cancer.

It wasn't the best time of my life.

And ironically, I had relished turning forty - I had gained a new-found confidence in my womanliness as I turned that milestone and finally felt like a grown-up, of sorts anyway.

By forty-one I was quite broken. Years of abandoning myself within my marriage was taking its toll. My husband was a soul mate in the truest sense of the word − here to help teach me lessons and for my soul to evolve, not in the light, love and fluffy kind of way that people often perceive soul mates, but in the dark, painful, deep, tough lessons sense.

Once we had separated, I was relieved to have my coil removed, looking forward to my body settling. There was a defiant sense of 'Fuck you, men, I can do without you' and sex with anyone else wasn't on the cards at the time − the last thing I wanted was another relationship. It also appeared to have become a physical impossibility for another coil to be put into place. It's not great, lying with your legs akimbo with a nurse excitedly calling her colleague over to 'take a look at this' whilst studying your most intimate feminine sanctuary. Apparently, a pinhole cervix is a rare sight to behold and studied.

"Er hello! I'm still here at the other end whilst you two are peering up into my yoni and getting all excited about its rarity."

And so along with the ending of my marriage, my relationship with the coil also came to a close, ignominiously marked with the words 'You'll never get another one in there'.

Having done copious amounts of research, I was definitely not entertaining the idea of going back on the pill… just in case I met a new man worthy of the delights of my possibly perimenopausal body and my pinhole cervix. I was already holding onto regrets about starting the pill at fifteen to try and cope with what I thought were heavy periods. Maybe they were, maybe they were normal, I have no idea and it's so long ago my memory has dismissed the full details. What I did know with the benefit of hindsight and wisdom was that years of messing around with my natural hormone balance was not a great idea even though mainstream medicine happily continues to encourage it as some kind of panacea for women.

My periods didn't return for almost a year after the coil was removed but the night sweats did settle down which was a real bonus. With a sigh of relief, I concluded I wasn't menopausal just yet, it was merely the coil running out of hormone juice. Well, that is what I chose to believe.

Like most marriage breakdowns, I found the time immensely stressful, I lost seven kilos in a matter of weeks, the tears seemed uncontrollable and never ending and my hair became really thin. I was a shadow of my former self and my poor body was expressing the hurt, the anger and the pain.

The body is the most intuitive and incredible guidance system, always reflecting on the outside whatever is going on within. When we take time to tune in and listen, to look deeper than the surface ailment or symptom, there will always be a message, emotions or experiences to heal and forgiveness to be considered.

There was much to heal. I was forty-one, barely any periods, no confidence, gaunt, unruly hair, two boys to love, support and nurture, a hobby business that wasn't going to keep the wolf from the door. It wasn't looking good yet somewhere almost imperceptible, was the smallest spark of flame burning within.

I had always been a highly independent young woman and I was yearning to rediscover that side of me again. I had a dream and desire for the freedom to live life on my terms, the opportunity to heal and I needed to know who I really was because by that point, I really had no idea. I was lost after years of conforming, trying to fit in and be the perfect mum, wife and party girl with a perfect body, clothes and conversation. On the outside I had done a pretty good job, the inside was not quite so.

As I became more stable and secure, my periods returned but they were exceptionally light (what a blessing) and quite irregular. I continued to think it was the after-effects of the coil. I was still too young for the menopause. My mum had a hysterectomy in her forties and we had never really discussed menopause so I didn't really have any maternal benchmark as to what age it might all happen for me.

What I did have on my side was my experience as a holistic therapist, particularly in reflexology. Most of my clients were ladies in their mid-years so I had researched menopause extensively even though I didn't apply my knowledge to my own experience initially. I was already a strong advocate of natural approaches and I instinctively knew about the innate wisdom of our bodies.

The average age for this momentous transition – if there is ever such a thing as a one size fits all average – is fifty-two apparently. You might be thirty-two or sixty-two. I had a client well into her sixties who was still bleeding every month, regular as clockwork – she wasn't particularly happy about that but when do we get to fully accept and love our body for all that it is? It is our home, our vessel of life yet it often takes us a lifetime to appreciate it.

Whilst I was highly skilled at guiding others through their journey, it took a long while to recognise my own experience. It wasn't until a few years later when I was in a new relationship and my periods had stopped completely for a few months that I really began to acknowledge and accept where I was at on my journey.

In average terms, I was still on the younger side of fifty and it had been such a gradual shift and evolution with no extremes of anything, unlike the transition I had expected. Menopause is like the antithesis to when we enter our menstrual years – the first period strikes like a meteor out of nowhere and then for the most part, there they are, a constant in life, month in, month out. Periods tend to have a definite start whereas the menopause has no defining moment, it is a time of easing off and fading with no start or stop point, it just morphs and becomes a way of life for several years. I trust it is perfect in its design as it gives us time to adjust emotionally and physically to this key metamorphosis.

Compared to many women, I would class myself as fortunate in my menopause experience. But I also have a theory that there might be more to it than just luck as menopause is heavily influenced by how we care for our body in the many years preceding, not just through the changing years.

We are a complex and intricately woven balance of body, mind and soul, the physical, mental and spiritual. Everything that we put into and onto our body has an impact on our delicate yet highly sophisticated system.

In my days of being a reflexologist, I helped many women with their menopausal symptoms, particularly hot flushes and night sweats. These women became regular clients, visiting every month for many years and for the most part I am sure their menopause was more manageable because of this treatment. Despite all my training, knowledge and understanding, the wonder of pressing on various points on the feet to create so much benefit in the body never ceased to amaze me

I remember one of my clients who was having a dire time, her night sweats were hot, soaking, clean sheets every night kind of events. The disturbed sleep, the impact on her husband and the consequent loathing of her body could not be underestimated. HRT wasn't agreeing with her and she was becoming depressed and disillusioned with life. A far too familiar story that millions of women experience as their menopause.

Yet her body would respond to reflexology in a consistent way – the following night or two after a treatment would always be worse, almost like an expulsion of symptoms and then the flushes would decrease significantly for a few days before increasing again. With regular treatment, the sweats became less and less, the HRT was abandoned, and life returned to a relatively enjoyable place to be. The body is amazing and yet sometimes it just needs some help to recalibrate which is exactly what reflexology and other energy therapies, do.

Since my training, I made sure that receiving a treatment was a regular part of my own self-care, practising what I preached and supporting my body through all the stresses of the outer world. I also went for many healing sessions after my marriage break up, having someone else moving energy through my body and holding a sacred space felt so necessary and cathartic.

The body is at its peak when it is in a state of homeostasis – one of equilibrium which is maintained by internal self-regulation – and it is beautifully engineered to do this when it is supported on every level.

However, life can make it pretty difficult to maintain this state!

Our hormonal, or endocrine system, is easily disrupted and I firmly believe that this is one of the reasons why the menopause experience is so different for everyone – our personal level of internal imbalances has a massive impact before we even begin with the hormone havoc of menopause.

Our hormones are affected by so many different things – stress being one of the biggest and most influential. For the vast majority of us, both men and women, we exist at best in a state of underlying, unacknowledged trickles of stress and at worst, dealing face-on with life-derailing situations. The natural response to stress is absolute genius in its creation and I make no apologies for this very brief biology lesson as the more we each take responsibility for understanding our body, the better equipped we are to support it.

When faced with a stressful situation, the adrenal glands release adrenaline, cortisol and a cascade of other hormones which impact the body and the brain. This chemical response is designed to give clarity so that you never have to ponder what to do in highly dangerous situations, you just react instinctively. The liver releases glucose into the muscles so that you can run or fight in the classic fight or flight stress response. The digestive system shuts down as your body doesn't want to use valuable resources digesting food in the moment of action and your sex hormones also switch off because let's face it, you really cannot be doing with distracting thoughts about sex in a moment of extreme danger. Just imagine being faced with a potential attack and you start to get distracted with lust and desire for the love of your life, it's just not appropriate.

After the danger has passed, the natural response is for the body to move into a place of collapse or release which helps restore the internal hormones and chemicals. This is why we feel extreme exhaustion or start trembling after facing danger and why animals shake, they are literally throwing off the excess chemical reaction. The stress response is perfectly designed for its original purpose. The problem is, we more often than not live in a permanent state of low-level stress – be it work, traffic, relationships, time pressure, finances, family, the world at large and so on – and whilst the body is continually responding to all of this, we are for the most part not releasing any of the excesses, leading instead to long standing accumulation of chemical and hormonal imbalance within this beautiful home in which we live.

Depending on what has happened in your life, you may have had twenty, thirty, forty years or an entire lifetime of stress response and chemical disruption bubbling around in your beautifully designed body. It is no wonder then, that by the time we reach this transition in menopause, it is not always an easy, comfortable or straightforward process. Our hormone balance is already vastly out of kilter and then suddenly the body is asking it to go through a massive reset – it's a big ask and just not the way we are designed to process this time.

This imbalance – and more specifically the role of cortisol, is also a fundamental contributor to the unwelcome accumulation of more fat around the waistline and thyroid issues which both tend to throw themselves into the mid-life party that is menopause. Not only do we have hot flushes, irregular periods, mood swings and a foggy brain to contend with, but we also have an expanding waist, fatigue and general sluggishness. It's hardly any wonder that menopause is a much-maligned phase of life.

And then there are the other bonuses, some of which casually strolled in with my burgeoning new relationship … the joys of vaginal dryness, painful sex and sagging – yes that is a thing. The vaginal muscles lose their tone and before you know it, a quick glance down reveals that your once pert pussy is now a little droopy. No one ever tells you about that. Or that low oestrogen can cause the skin to thin and tear. Or that your vagina can actually shrink … or stretch. Maybe it's better that no one forewarns you, at least the lack of knowledge is one less thing to worry about! Ironically at the time of your life when you may feel least like sex or masturbation despite having a risk-free pass, the best thing for your vaginal health and natural lubrication is to actually use it more. Much as I marvel constantly at the incredible design of the body, I think some aspects of the creative process were a Friday afternoon or Monday morning job.

But I digress.

The finely tuned internal body is one of the reasons why I believe that it is the many years preceding the pause that play such a key role in our experience.

If that's so, you might question how I had it so easy when I been through such huge stress in the years leading up to my own menopause experience and stress is such a biggie in symptoms. To counter the stress, I had started working more with energy and healing and dedicating time to keeping my body in balance. Meditation was a regular feature of my week – I say week because it certainly wasn't daily, I was receiving reflexology or a head massage at least monthly and exercise was a fundamental part of my routine. All of which support the body to move from sympathetic dominance (the stressed, high alert, all systems go function) into parasympathetic (the rebalancing, relaxing and restoring phase). I wasn't the model of healthy perfection or without vices by any means and I was partial to a few glasses of wine, however there were some good solid basics in place.

Whatever stage of the menopausal transition you are at, it is never too late to introduce practices to help you and the more you can encourage your nervous system into a state of deep relaxation, inner calm and balance, the more it will benefit your overall health as well as your menopause experience.

Obviously, the earlier we start supporting ourselves physically and emotionally, the better. And if we can teach and encourage our daughters and younger women about the lifelong effects of self-care, what a different we can make to generations going forward. Wouldn't it be wonderful if the vast majority of women of the future could for the most part embrace and revel in their menopause, to appreciate it for its process and experience it more easily, lovingly and holistically – I live in hope for it to be this way.

As women we tend to spend much of our lives putting our own needs at the bottom of the list. There is an endemic belief that has evolved through centuries of patriarchal rule, which means taking time for ourselves is selfish. With the rise of the feminist movement and the striving to be all things equal to all men, we have as a collective tended to suppress our needs even further as we compete in the workplace whilst often still holding on to the traditional role of being the linchpin within the home. Clearly this is not the case for every woman but taking a broad sweep across society, it is often so.

All too often, the price we have paid for 'having it all' is of putting our personal needs and desires way down on the priority list when in all honesty, we deserve to be at right at the top. Only when we fully nourish ourselves, emotionally, physically and spiritually, are we truly in a place to nurture all those around us, to give everyone the best and fullest version of ourselves rather than the depleted, exhausted and run-ragged all-things-to-all-people version. Giving myself the gift of time and space to truly relax has been a game changer in terms of my relationships with my partner, my family and my business and I have become really comfortable with being selfish about my needs. I remember as a teenager my parents made me join a youth club as I supposedly spent too much time on my own but as it transpires, dammit I was very happy in my own company and it was actually really good for me.

Suffice to say if you are in constant people-pleasing mode, never say no and your nervous system is firing up all the time, even whilst you are supposedly doing something for yourself it becomes counter-productive. Taking a bath and running through the shopping list in your mind, worrying about your business or using the bath simply as a tick off your to do list (yes, yes, I've ticked self-care off the list for today) quickly evaporates the benefit and becomes a wasted opportunity of truly nourishing yourself, your body and your energy.

When was the last time you gave yourself permission to fully relax and do something just for you? If it's been a while, make a promise to start today – it might not come easily but your body will love it. And if you are going to pamper yourself do read on before you jump into that luxurious bath ….as the other great disruptor of our delicate body chemistry is the chemical toxins we ingest, inhale and slather ourselves in.

With the dissolution of my marriage and the blossoming of the true me, there came a much deeper reconnection with my inner witch, the part of me that has existed for many lifetimes, the piece of my soul that remembered old wisdom, how to heal using nature and her gifts, the magic of Mother Earth and of greater consciousness. And with that ancient knowing stirring, I started to look more into natural alternatives as a means of caring for my physical body. What I learned was both disturbing and enlightening.

It is well documented that for much of the modern world, our drinking water is laden with chemicals and hormones. The advent of the pill and its mass usage has led to significant quantities of oestrogen filtering into our water supply which can logically only serve to create imbalances within all of us. Is it any worder that since the common use of the pill, we are beginning to see more people identifying with different genders, being born into the 'wrong' body, the advent of man boobs, periods starting younger and the rise in breast cancers? And shit menopauses.

Water is also just a drop in the ocean of contaminants. Food has vast quantities of chemicals and toxins from the copious amounts of routinely sprayed herbicides and pesticides which sneak their way into the body and its internal make up. It is not without the deepest irony that one of my first jobs was working for a petrochemical company that produced those very chemicals that I am now so vehemently against. Life is always a learning.

And then we have skincare. My goodness we put some toxic crap onto our skin. To put the impact of skincare chemicals into some perspective – and so you might begin to understand a tiny bit of my soapbox passion for this subject - according to research, the average woman applies around five hundred chemicals to her body every day, sixty per cent of which are absorbed into the skin. Five hundred per day over the course of a year is 182,500. Let's assume that these average starts accumulating from the age of sixteen, that's almost 5.5 million by the time we reach forty-six!

5.5 million! And from that, 3.3 million may well have crept into your body.

So, whilst the chemists and scientists happily claim that all these chemicals are safe and cause no harm, from my perspective, the accumulative impact speaks a very different story.

Many of the key ingredients in soaps, shower or bath wash, shampoo, conditioner, moisturiser, mascara, foundation, perfume and sunscreen (plus everything else!) are well recognised to mimic hormones once in the body, more specifically oestrogen. Parabens (and there's a big family of them) are a form of preservative commonly used in all kinds of personal and home care products which are widely known for disrupting and behaving like hormones once in the body.

Our beautifully balanced inner chemistry is systematically being disrupted for years way before we even begin to approach menopause, so it really is no great surprise that it has become such an ordeal for so many.

My theory of an easier menopause is that the elimination of as many toxins as possible from my food, my home and my skincare in the preceding years all combined to play a really key role in my relatively easy experience. By reducing the toxins that mimic hormones in the body, which has served me, and my body well. I will admit there have been days when I have had stinky armpits (my trialling of natural deodorants took a while!) and I no longer waft into a room in a haze of parfum or product-styled hair but the payoff for a less explosive menopause has been well worth it.

We are now blessed with a much higher awareness and greater choice although I would add a note of caution that some manufacturers are pretty clever with their branding – just because a label has the word 'Natural', is adorned with pretty flowers and leaves, or advertises a certain natural ingredient, it does not by any stretch of the imagination guarantee that the product is free from toxic additives. It can be a labour of love to commit to learning about ingredients and reading the ingredient list on packaging – especially with the failing vision that besets most of us around the menopause years! I am forever fishing for my reading glasses in my bag so that I can read the miniscule print on a label detailing the ingredients – my shopping trips can be lengthy.

Most importantly, it is never too late to start making changes, however big or small. Every little step you take to remove chemicals, toxins and stress will support your body, long term health and your menopause experience. Even if you are post menopause, it can only be of benefit. Buy organic when you can (check out the Dirty Dozen if you want to know where to start), substitute personal care products for more natural alternatives and reduce stress whenever you can … your body will love you for every step you take. And your body is where you live longest after all.

THE MENOPAUSAL MIND

The body and mind are inextricably linked, they are not separate things that work independently of each other. The design of the human is far too complex and advanced for such basics. Our cells respond to our thoughts, feelings and emotions which actually means we are the most incredible and powerful beings when we can harness the mind. And that is one hell of a tricky road to navigate during the peri and menopause years.

Depression jumps in out of nowhere and normal brain function is often a distant memory. Finding your handbag in the fridge can seem perfectly normal as can staring at your best friend and having no idea what her name is. I've lost count of the number of times I have seemingly lost my manners for not introducing someone simply because the names have temporarily vanished into thin air. How can I literally be looking at someone and have no idea what they are called? I suppose this is matched only by my mum at my wedding asking my long since divorced dad who he was!

Learning to master the mind is an ongoing project for all of humanity. The more we understand our internal world, the easier it is to create a reality that is easier, more harmonious and feels good.

After my husband and I separated, I frequently felt that I had lost my mind completely. Whilst I had been the love of his life and placed on a pedestal, given flowers every week and wanted for nothing financially, I was also under a spell of control, conditions and conformity. And that just intensified once I was no longer his. He struggled to cope with my freedom, the fact that I was surviving on my own and that I was moving on.

There were so many head fuck moments (there is no other word to describe what was happening in my mind) when I didn't know if something was real or imagined. I was convinced my house was bugged, I was pretty sure I was being followed by a private detective and there were countless incidences and injustices which made me as mad as hell. I didn't (and still don't) think any of this was perimenopausal irrationality, it was way too real. But maybe it was related to my hormones too. When we are stuck in something, it's really hard to see the situation with clarity.

Many times, I thought I was going crazy to the point that I didn't physically know what to do with myself but I soon learnt to choose to rise to the bait and get angry or let things go over my head as much as possible. And letting things go was exactly what I did for my own sanity and for the sake of making life as easy as possible for my boys. My mum and dad had split up when I was four and they were at war pretty much until my wedding day … and that wasn't something I wanted my boys to experience. I wanted them to have divorced parents who could behave like adults, communicate and show that there was still an element of care. For the love of God that was hard sometimes!

'Breeeeaaaathe Su breathe. Let it go. It's not worth it. Don't give it your time or energy' became one of my regular mantras.

Age, wisdom and menopause do come with many gifts, one of which is being able to look more objectively and take decisions based on what is best for me. Because ultimately, my life is all about me. Much as your life is all about you. That's not selfish, it is ultimate self-care. I'm not saying my approach of letting go was easy, but it worked for me. The more I practised, the easier it became. And it was actually way easier than getting angry and constantly feeling hurt, bitter and emotionally battered.

The longer we hold on to any thoughts or feelings that don't serve us, the more they become ingrained and create dis-ease. An unhappy or toxic mind crates toxicity in the body which leads to illness, pain or stress ....and it doesn't help the whole menopause process either. A calm and peaceful mind is like an oasis within the self and the body cannot help but respond. So many of us are not raised to really love who we are or even to like or be kind to ourselves. We give ourselves a tough time over and over yet what is the purpose of that? It doesn't do us any good on any level so let's just call a stop to it now. And let's make a pact to help raise young people to accept that self-love is the greatest thing we can ever give ourselves – what a very different world we would all be living in if that was our normal self-perception. I wish I had learnt to love myself from childhood.

And I would lay money on the fact that we would all be having better menopauses if we had already spent a lifetime loving ourselves.

Eventually, I came to a point with my ex-husband where in all my choices about how to respond, I finally chose to forgive. Forgiveness is a truly powerful process on every level, mentally, emotionally and spiritually. Forgiveness isn't about condoning; it is about setting yourself and the other person free. I forgave him for all the hurtful words he had spoken, for the control and manipulation, the countless times when sex had been forced upon me and all the moments when my needs had been swept aside. I did it for me. I just let it all go

And it was really good, way more than good for my mind, my heart and my soul.

I also realised that I had to forgive myself for the part I had played, it's never just a one-way street. I had abandoned myself over and over. I had allowed myself to ignore my intuition, I had failed to stand up for my needs or to simply stand my ground full stop. I had been so determined to be a nice, good woman; I had put out my own fire as much as he had extinguished it. I had to recognise my role and accept it – and that wasn't easy because it was far easier to blame someone else than take a deep hard look at myself and my faults.

After years, just like putting down heavy bags of shopping that I had been carrying around for eons, I became light and free

It meant that he could no longer hurt me because there was nothing there to hurt. I was fully back to myself, taking responsibility for my emotions and responses. That is the magic of menopause as we grasp that new commitment to who we truly are. Why would I continue letting someone else dictate my feelings, directly or indirectly – I would never win that battle. Forgiveness also meant that I could sit by his side, hold his hand and stroke his head when the larger-than-life bon viveur finally lost his battle with alcohol, ending a cycle of life together from a place of love and compassion and nothing else. Soul mates give us interesting journeys.

Alongside this letting go, I started to dig deeper into my mind the more I moved through the menopause. Meditation remained a key part of my life and I started journaling regularly as it was an effective way of unloading the hard times I was frequently giving myself (and oh my goodness, I could give myself such a tough time) and then processing my thoughts. I began to unravel myself in a positive and empowering way rather than a dishevelling... although there were definitely moments of messiness, tears and snot because when we begin a process of rebirth, there has to be a clearing too. Much like most women cannot give birth without pooping, we cannot birth into our third age without releasing some of the mental and emotional shit and congestion out of the way first. Or I guess we can just keep our legs crossed forever in abject refusal to let go, we always have choices.

The more I have shed mentally and emotionally, the easier it has become to speak my mind and be truthful. From the child who never put her hand up in class to the young woman who would virtually vomit at the thought of doing a presentation or speaking to any more than five people to the mid-fifty something who knows that it is way more important to speak my truth and share my words than to keep them silent.

One of the greatest things about menopause is that we begin to care less about what others think of us and more about being true to ourselves. Our brain switches from people pleasing and politeness to a 'Fuck that!' I am just going to be myself attitude. The mind becomes less entrapped by other people's opinions and clearer on the concept 'What is right for me becomes right for everyone'. What a sacrilege of life if we don't embrace this.

When we care for the mind, we care for the body. And as with the body, it is never too late to start. We are mind, body and soul.

THE EVOLUTION OF THE SOUL

Menopause always used to be referred to as 'The Change', usually in hushed whispers as if it were a terrible affliction that only certain women went through. I can hear the words in my teenage memory, 'Ssssh, be careful, she's going through the change, poor thing' as if any menopausal woman might turn into a loose cannon (ok, sometimes we do!) or implode on touch. I have no idea when that terminology ceased to be used but we cannot deny that it is most certainly a change of life – physically, emotionally and spiritually.

The spiritual side of menopause is an opportunity for a deep reconnection with self but often a recognition that there is more to us than just the physical body. We start to face our own mortality with a little more realism, to notice how the years have flown by and perhaps to question the purpose of our soul in the human form.

It is a time when we begin to ask pertinent and more inquiring questions, often because for the first time in our adult lives we actually start to have time to focus on the I.

Who am I really?

What am I here for?

What do I want to do with my life?

What are my real dreams and ambitions?

What is the legacy I want to leave?

How can I feel more fulfilled and complete?

My menopause came with many questions. This is our time to truly live life on our terms. In some ways it feels like the last big chance we get although in reality we are often only two thirds or even half way through our life when menopause appears. My grandmother lived to 105 so I reckon I could well be only half way... But we never know how long we have so it becomes vitally important that we live in the now and live in a way that serves us on every single level.

Our soul comes into this human body with lessons to learn, experiences to gain and old wounds to heal. We often hit menopause and realise that so much of our life has not really been serving us on a soul level – perhaps the job, or the relationship, the friends or patterns of behaviour. We begin to question who we really are, what we are here for and suddenly have the desire to make momentous changes. It isn't a mid-life crisis, it's a liberation and finally an honouring of the soul, throwing off all the 'shoulds' and conditions that we have been attached to and grasping that wonderful opportunity to become the fullest expression of who we are. If not now, when?

In pagan traditions, menopause signified women moving into the role of the crone – not a term most of us now relish thanks to the patriarchal demonisation of women which has led to the current definitions of hag, old bag, witch and ugly old woman – is it no wonder society misaligns this incredible phase of our life so much?

The word crone originally derived from the word for crown and the top of the head is where our crown chakra is positioned, the seat of our connection to higher consciousness (chakras are vortexes of energy that run through our body as well as above and below, the key seven are positioned along the spine). On a spiritual level, moving into our crown or crone phase is where women traditionally became recognised for their wisdom, for being the wise elders and teachers and receiving greater acknowledgement for their femininity and natural beauty. The crown chakra is said to only develop fully and open at the age of forty-nine (a little later for men!) and this may well be why we become more intuitive, spiritually connected, and conversant with our higher self around the same time as we transition into menopause.

We are wise by this point. Far wiser than we often know or acknowledge. We may have created new life. We have years of experiences, learnings and emotions to share. And now by a dint of nature, we get the chance to recognise it all.

As the womb ceases to be a practical creatrix of life, we are gifted the opportunity to reconnect with this powerful portal within us. The womb is far more than an empty space where we grow babies. It is a truly magical place where we hold infinite space and energy for receiving and creating. We have been blessed with the most incredible gift of being able to bring new humans into the world and to hold this source of infinite power, yet for so many of us, this space becomes forgotten, dismissed or a source of despair. The womb represents a microcosm of the whole universe and menopause is an invitation for us to step into the centre of this, to become the centre of our own world as well as of the universe and existence itself. How flipping incredible is that? How blessed are we as women to be given such a gift that exists within us?

The true nature of menopause has been suppressed and denied from us for hundreds if not thousands of years yet now we are beginning to re-remember what an opportunity it is for spiritual growth and evolution of the soul.

We enter into this life form in the womb. We leave through the crown. The crone phase is a long-forgotten welcoming of pure magic and potential.

As I have moved through menopause, I have certainly developed a deep relationship with God, the Universe, Consciousness, One - the name is just a name and whatever resonates with each of us personally. It is a very separate thing to religion, it is a sense of a higher consciousness within me and around me and it is uplifting, loving and powerful. And the more I allow this energy of the Divine Masculine in, the softer yet stronger I become.

Whatever our gender, we are in harmony when we are in energetic balance, the yin and yang, the masculine and feminine. This balance, like so many elements, represents two opposites that can only exist together, like night and day, dark and light, heaven and earth. As above, so below, as within, so without.

We all embody both masculine and feminine energies and these have nothing to do with gender or sex, they are simply energies. The masculine energy is very much our state of doing, taking action, making things happen and it is also the energy of providing. The feminine balance is our state of BEing, creativity, inner guidance and our ability to receive. As women, we have become very accustomed to spending a lot of time in our masculine and very little in the feminine, creating a spiritual and energetic disconnect, particularly with our womb space.

Embracing this balance has probably been the most challenging part of my third age. I have had to learn to allow myself to be supported, to be vulnerable and open and to stop being so damn independent. It's a strength to let all of this in, not a weakness. It comes from a place of inner connection and trust in myself, not from a place of victimhood or helplessness.

And it is a beautiful place to be.

Menopause could and should be an incredible experience for all women. A returning to ourselves, a reconnection with our true power and an embracing of our wisdom and ability to teach. There are many wonderful and positive aspects to menopause and the more we can return to our natural state of being, our innate feminine wisdom and inner harmony in the physical, mental and spiritual realms, the easier and more fulfilling the whole experience can be.

It is time for women to learn once again to embrace and relish the journey.

Reflections

Reflections

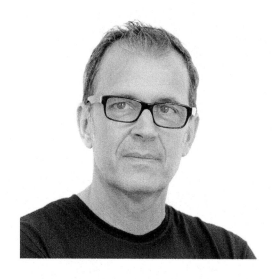

NEIL USHER
UK

Neil Usher has been solving complex real estate, workplace and change problems for over thirty years, blending straightforward and creative thinking with an eye for both strategy and detail. His global experience in both corporate and advisory roles spans a variety of industry sectors. His projects have won multiple awards, and he is widely regarded as a leading practitioner in his field.

Neil has been actively blogging about work, the workplace and change for over a decade and has authored a book on each. He is a sought-after conference and academic speaker, always bringing a fresh perspective while challenging assumptions and myths.

That said, he prefers to be thought of as 'a regular bloke just trying to make sense of it all.'

You can read more of Neil's work here https://workessence.medium.com

Chapter Five

PUTTING THE MEN IN MENOPAUSE

Men don't have a menopause. It follows that we don't know about it, think about it or write about it. Where we see or find ourselves on the receiving end of the effects of the menopause in a woman, we most often attribute another cause entirely, sourced from a diminutive catalogue. Where none inevitably fit, a character flaw suffices, an inability to get a grip. The menopause is, after all, a woman's issue. Theirs to anticipate, bear, understand and overcome. We have enough to deal with.

We might. Only we have no biologically defined life phases beyond puberty. That makes it both simple and complex. Simple in that there's nothing to anticipate; complex in that conscious changes of physiology, perspective or persona are rarely attributable or explicable. Women have two clearly demarcated phases. The first, around thirty years from puberty to menopause, the second post-menopause till close. The same woman, but not the same woman in each.

During the first phase, while women are enjoying the relatively contained and well-documented inconvenience of the menstrual cycle interspersed with the bearing and delivering of children, as men we're primarily concerned with whether we can still get it up. There is a lot riding on it. Or, at least, we hope there will be. The male road stretches in glorious perpendicularity from the breaking of the voice to a hazy horizon where nothing works anymore. Which means, unlike women, we're starting from a position where significant life events are manufactured, not given. It's a key point of difference we need to grasp.

There is of course the over-entitled tantrum that is the 'mid-life crisis' (a term coined by psychoanalyst Elliott Jacques in 1965) where, in a desperate attempt to rediscover a virility cruelly eroded by two decades of overwhelming responsibility and self-denial, we embark on a documentary-worthy journey in (or on) a suitably impractical item of personal transport. Or at least run it through our mind as a possibility, if we wanted to. It's often prompted by an awareness that time has taken its toll on earlier ambitions and aspirations, exacerbated by the regret associated with not having pursued other options when they presented themselves, or with a little more application effort may have done so. Yet while it's a term in popular use, often to justify incidences of poor behaviour, evidence suggests that the actuality is uncommon. As is often discovered, too, its medical half-brother, erectile disfunction, is rarely resolved in the pursuit of a morally-bankrupt coast-to-coast. We're just saddled with it, looking for a scapegoat.

Much amusement is derived societally from our misguided and failed attempts to 'understand women.' That is, principally because we focus on outcome rather than cause. The latter would reveal that we need to understand women twice. The menopause, poised between the first and second phase of a woman's life, is not just an event in itself to comprehend, which is how it's often positioned, but is vital to an appreciation of the difference between the two phases. Applying a model of the first to the second – or vice versa – can be disastrous. If the menopause is a mystery to us, naturally so will be the two phases. This level of what can only be described as ignorance has no place in modern society. We can do so much better.

Somewhat surprisingly, though, the menopause is something of a mystery to many women, too. Either in being not researched prior to its occurrence, or because despite an increase in media attention in the last five years, they don't like to talk about it when it's happening. Certainly not to us. There remains a genuine fear of negative judgment – from men and women alike – from owning up to being in its throes, for two key reasons. First, for the fact that it signals the end of a woman's fertility, and in many minds therefore, usefulness. Second, for the perception of the woman being beset by, and inevitably unable to manage, a plethora of unpleasant symptoms. To a degree therefore, if women aren't admitting to or talking about their menopause, what chance do we stand of learning? Given our tendency to try and wriggle out of jail free, there's an up-and-over garage door of an exit.

It's worth remembering that our understanding at any depth is fairly recent, despite the fact that Aristotle mentioned it (but then he mentioned most things), due to changes in life expectancy. As late as 1900 in the UK the average age at which a woman slipped off this mortal coil was fifty. Which meant that for many women, they didn't get as far as a menopause, and if they did, they'd often had so many children, given our right to irresponsible, consequence-free sexual fulfilment, that it was hard to separate the causal threads of bodily brokenness.

As a final opening clarification, a word in regard to gender identification. The menopause is a biological fact. If you have ovaries, at the appropriate time you'll have a menopause. However, you identify. It's just the way it is.

With the understanding we now have of the menopause – its causes, effects, mitigations and opportunities – it's hoped that this chapter will constitute all a man needs to read to begin to build a picture of not just the menopause in isolation and how they can positively help at this time, but of a woman's life overall. If you've got this far, clear the decks for half an hour and see it through.

THE EVENTS

We begin with an essential caveat. I'm not a medically qualified practitioner. Possibly merely a moderately medically aware citizen. My wife is a menopause coach, and the house has a lot of books on the subject. Including hers, which during its development and drafting we shared facts, ideas and perspectives. While I learned a lot, she's the expert. Yet there's a world of misinformation out there that butts right up against preposterous conspiracy, and I wouldn't wish to inadvertently add to it. It's advisable therefore to conduct your own research and validate (or not) what follows.

As mentioned, the menopause sits between the two phases of womanhood, both of which have remarkably thus far managed to arrive without a name other than 'first' (from puberty to the menopause) and 'second' (which begins when the menopause is over). And even these terms are rarely used. Quite a brand fail. We'll say more about them in due course.

The name 'menopause' is used to cover a period of four-eight years which usually begins around age forty-five. Let's not forget, most women of forty-five look younger than forty in keeping with a progressively greater focus on wellbeing. The media, who in recent years have begun opening themselves to the existence of the menopause, often don't help. They portray menopausal women as in their sixties and seventies, beyond their usefulness, for whom pasture is the only viable habitat. They know better. They should do so much better.

The entirety consists of the 'perimenopause' or the warm-up act, the main event, and the warm-down. It eases in, happens, and eases out. It's here we start to get used the approximations, uncertainty and unpredictability that characterise the entire experience.

It's essentially all about eggs. A woman has around a million of them at birth as a starter pack, stored in her ovaries. They're already down to 300,0000 by puberty. As a finite resource, they continue to decline in number thereafter. That's nothing compared to the 525 billion sperm we produce over our lifetime. We don't take any chances. As the decline in egg production nears its conclusion, the production of the three hormones that play a vital role in the reproductive cycle, testosterone (yes, the one that we thrive on), oestrogen and progesterone, falls to a level that causes menopausal symptoms to begin.

Somewhere within these four-eight years is the twelve-month event – the *actual* menopause – from the woman's last period to *exactly* one year later, after which she is no longer fertile. Pregnancy is a physical impossibility. The eggs are discontinued and hormone production reverts to pre-pubescent levels. Which isn't very much at all.

The date of the last period is not clear cut. The woman may go for eleven and a half months without one and then have to hunt in the attic for the tampons, in which case the clock starts all over again. So, the logistics for the big all-in full-on cycle-free celebration party can be tricky. Symptoms continue post-menopause until at an indeterminate point, they subside. They may never entirely vanish.

The menopause for every woman is as unique as a fingerprint. Unpredictability comes as standard. For eight years. That's around a tenth of a lifetime, over a fifth of a career. We worry that a common cold lasts a fortnight. In a world where we like to instantly identify an issue and its fix through a helpful YouTube clip, this is beyond problematic. We know at this stage there's stuff that's going to happen, with an approximate arrival date and timescale. We now need to consider what will happen, and how.

THE SYMPTOMS

Our desire for certainty and specificity is challenged by the menopause. We need to consider there are forty symptoms. A quite staggering range. We can probably name two or three, at best. They vary in frequency and magnitude for the duration. They will arrive and leave at various times. Some will trigger others.

Most symptoms will have at least one other potential cause that is not menopause-related that may require investigation and disproval. When struggling to identify the cause of the visible or invisible symptoms being experienced, there isn't a 'pee stick' from the pharmacy that will indicate what it is, it has to be pieced together. Symptoms are very often hidden or downplayed, so we're not even entirely sure they're there at all. It makes diagnosis spurious at first. Very often other possibilities require investigation and disproval.

Age is usually a giveaway, or at least a reason to suspect. Yet most women believe themselves too young to be perimenopausal, given the media grey-wash. Women are so often prescribed anti-depressants it's the modern equivalent of being carted off to the asylum for being deemed hysterical. Help generally needs to be fought or paid for.

The symptoms are, at a rudimentary level, both physical and psychological. It's interesting that very few are exclusively female in nature, as in they relate to a woman's physiology alone. In fact, there are only two – breast pain ('moobs' – common in men of this age – are excluded) and vaginal dryness. As for the overwhelming majority, men can and do suffer isolated incidences of each. In which instances we usually ensure everyone gets to hear all about it. So, while they occur to women at the time of the menopause, they're not 'women's issues.'

A rundown of the symptoms is shown below:

PHYSICAL	PSYCHOLOGICAL
Allergies	Anxiety
Breast Pain	Depression
Brittle nails	Difficulty concentrating
Changes in body odour	Loss of Confidence
Cold Flushes	Loss of sex drive
Digestive problems	Loss of verbal recall
Dizziness	Memory Lapses
Dry hair	Mood swings
Dry skin	Panic Attacks
Fatigue	
Flooding	
Gum problems	
Hair loss	
Hot flushes	
Incontinence (stress and urge)	
Insomnia	
Irregular periods	
Itchy skin – formication	
Joint pain	
Loss of muscle mass	

Migraines

Night Sweats

Recurrent UTIs

Sleep Apnoea

Snoring

Stiff joints

Thrush (increased susceptibility)

Tinnitus

Unwanted hair growth

Weight gain

Vaginal atrophy/dryness

The trouble with a list is that every items just looks like an item on a list, which gives no indication of relative impact or scale. Anxiety can have devastating and wide-ranging effects. Snoring is just annoying for anyone in earshot. Unless it's keeping a partner awake who has a critical job and whose performance begins to suffer with negative consequences for those with who they are in contact. Every symptom tells its own story.

Certain symptoms are triggers for others. They're not neatly packaged modules. Digestive problems may contribute to a lack of sleep, which in turn causes or exacerbates mood swings and fluctuations in concentration. Similarly, depression and loss of confidence may result from hair loss and fatigue. The relationship between symptoms is dynamic and complex.

THE LOCATIONS

There are three areas in which these symptoms will rage, in which men will experience their direct and referred effect and have a choice as to how to respond.

Menopause at home

In principle, home should be the easiest arena in which to be open and clear about the menopause. A closed environment in which everyone knows everyone, and each has probably seen the others naked and sat astride the lavatory too many times to mention. Of course, not every domestic environment is this free of inhibition and restraint. But all the same, it's generally a lot more so than work. Unless we're in adult entertainment.

Generally, we're talking partners and children, occasionally elderly dependents. Many women have had to face the stony silence of a mother in denial or refusal, as for the previous generation the menopause simply didn't happen. Which meant fathers didn't know about it or talk about it, either. They simply watched in disbelief – sometime anger – as their wives fell apart. They always had the pub in which to bemoan it. Which often meant danger after closing time. Our fathers never put their hand on our juvenile shoulder in the relieved silence after an unexpected maternal bollocking and said "Son, it's time we talked about the menopause."

For young children of course, accustomed to their mother being a source of stability, reliability, and unconditional love and care, the physical and emotional unpredictability that ensues can cause anxiety and fear. They need either parent to intervene and explain. Not with a medical manual, but a story, a metaphor, a representation they can understand depending on their age. It could be us that's called on to do this. We have to be ready.

Which leads us to the modern man. Aware, sensitive, strong, supportive and understanding. Reliable and yet impulsive. Serious and fun. Successful, yet humble. Not us? While much is expected of men within the family and without, the menopause rarely features among the challenges we'll face on our ascent to greatness. Because it's not ours, naturally. We're expected to be at the birth (occasionally the conception), the carol concert and the graduation. But not the breakdown.

The first time I told a group of friends that my wife was pursuing a career as a menopause coach, they stuffed their hands in their pockets, looked at the floor, shuffled and sniggered. It was, apparently, all too difficult. In all probability their partners were already at base camp.

Educated, articulate men in stable relationships with families, but not available. It was quite a realisation. There are no conditions precedent for our being there for our partner through the menopause. Sharing a home is no guarantee of our support.

Menopause at work

Work creates complex power relations. We often face three ways at once – upwards (our boss), sideways (our peers) and down (our team). There's much at stake in a career: finance, security and status amongst others. Whether physically co-located or at the end of a web call, agendas play out in both overt and obvious and covert and subtle ways. Sometimes the threat comes from what we can see, sometimes from what we can't.

With forty symptoms come forty subjects for the most enduring, ubiquitous and depressing bi-product of people brought together to work – 'banter.' Fed by prejudice of many forms and perpetrated mainly (but not exclusively) by men, it has quite incredibly for many decades been defended as harmless fun, principally by those contributing to it. Yet there is almost always a living, breathing object of ridicule.

While thankfully significant strides have been made in holding those responsible to account in several areas of prejudice – in particular with race – menopause often sits outside the parameters of justice. Which means that aside from simply trying to understand and deal with the complex and potentially debilitating nature of menopausal symptoms, there is the added problem of humiliation for either exhibiting them or raising the matter of suffering from them. For all the recent progress, menopause still has a validity problem as a debilitating condition. In many eyes it remains merely a weakness, the mocking of which is permissible.

Hot flushes, hair loss, weight gain, memory loss, panic attacks and mood swings offer ample subject matter for those intent on deflecting from their own physical and character inadequacies and self-directed deterioration. For deflection it often is. An admission of being menopausal doesn't remove the invitation, either, often inflating the target. Which is why so often such an admission never comes and the cloak is thrown. Women don't just leave the workplace because of the difficulty of dealing with their symptoms, but because of the way they are treated, too.

Yet aside from being remorselessly derided with no prospect of redress, there is also fear of the career damage the menopause may cause. Prejudice silently stalks deliberations of opportunity and reward. Can a woman who has become menopausal be trusted with key client relationships, negotiations, presentations, team building, all the stuff of management and leadership? What if she floods just as the contract is about to be signed? Best entrust someone younger. And male.

It's a difficult position to reconcile with the notion of 'psychological safety,' a thirty-year-old somewhat cumbersome academic expression that describes a situation within a team or group where we are able to express ideas, perspectives and concerns without fear of judgment or negative consequence. It's a situation in which everyone should find themselves at work, regardless. The admission of personal vulnerability has been claimed to contribute positively to collective team or group cohesion and performance. Yet it requires wholesale participation. Without it, fractures are exploited by those for whom personal interest is paramount. For men, whose moral compass serves as nothing more than a beermat, it remains a gilded gift horse. They can exchange a minor or trivial difficulty, and the upper hand is secured.

Menopause in love

It would be easy to accept or even talk up some menopausal symptoms as they relate to a love life. A little more curvaceous weight, skin-tingling sweat, even vaginal dryness (not just valued but instigated in some cultures). But that's the top-shelf offer (not that the internet has shelves, as such). In almost every respect, however, the menopause plays havoc with the corporate talent twins, attraction and retention. It's a churned field of barbed wire and imminent danger. If there are hidden cracks in a relationship, the menopause will reveal them.

We'll need to consider the menopause in two respects – within established relationships and for those seeking new.

Within established relationships, the menopause often emerges at a time of re-appraisal. Children have left home or are beginning to become self-reliant. A little freedom is returning. The years of parenting have all but erased the frizzle of desire that gave rise to them. The seemingly impossible opportunity to re-establish a relationship comprising both sex *and* responsibility emerges. Both parties consciously and subconsciously review – we've changed, is this the person I want to be with? Just as the woman's involuntary loss of interest in any form of intimacy lands.

Everything appears to be moving negatively, at a time when the reverse is called for. At this stage in our life, we're able to trade on our maturity – we exude sophistication, success, an easy calm. Assuming we haven't abandoned our self-respect entirely. In women these traits are often interpreted – by women and men alike – as intensity, arrogance, aloofness. Distinguished men are haggard women. Experience in men – charming, reassuring and alluring – is unprincipled looseness in women. Sluttishness even.

We place an undue value on freshness, while celebrating our own lack of it. All of which is sewn, fed and watered by both the arts and media. The passing male teenage fantasy about an 'older woman' is, let's not forget, targeted at someone in their late twenties or thirties. For MILF read YMILF. It's all relative.

We're simple creatures. We have a model and everything needs to fit within it. A loss of libido and vaginal dryness are because she's not turned on by us anymore, despite *all the effort* we're making. We can't do anything right. We're living on eggshells. We feel rejected. When faced with a sudden and withering barrage of symptoms, as the victim, electing to pursue other options, unburdened by the menopause (at least, for the time being) becomes increasingly attractive. Of the 525 billion accomplished swimmers there's a still a hell of a lot left, primed and ready. The world needs them far more than we do. It's all about us, after all. And so, we respond in the natural way – *we* reject.

That's problematic enough where a relationship already exists. For a woman attempting to begin and develop a relationship where none presently exists, it's even more daunting. "Fat, sweaty, moody insomniac seeks solvent, caring partner for fun and romance. NS. GSOH. Pets allowed." We're unlikely to be impressed even if the description is implicit rather than declared. An initial encounter has as much chance of developing into any form of maturity as a baby turtle hatched in the dunes with the salty ocean is its nostrils.

In every respect, therefore, it's no surprise that the highest suicide rates amongst women in the western hemisphere are those in their fifties, driven by the sense that it's really not worth hanging around when no-one considers you useful for anything anymore. Men are key to reversing this hugely disturbing trend. Yet for all the opportunities they have, we repeatedly hear that it takes a 'particular' type of man. Which is both deflating and dangerous.

Each of us should – and can – be of this particular type. There's no suggestion that this is an exercise in transforming the male into the 'modern man,' however appealing that might be. It's specific and focussed. If it leads to being so in other areas of life, that would be a bonus. For the rest of this essay, we'll explore how.

BEING THERE (AND DOING SOMETHING)

There's something intrinsically safe and reassuring for men about structure. Personally, I'm obsessed with it. E-mails, reports, presentations, talks, a framework where they start and end. The proposed approach to the menopause for men is simple, balanced and workable. There are three key and related areas of focus, four if we are in a relationship, which drive action and to which we can return if unsure.

As previously mentioned, this is not a medical, psychological or coaching perspective, it is driven by experience and (un)common sense. No qualifications are required to enter, and none are awarded on the way out.

Being there and doing something matters because it's the right thing to do. This isn't about 'return on investment' (ROI) or making life easier at the receiving end of the menopause. Neither is it a hack, a quick fix.

It's a long-term investment in being a better human being. It's a positive contribution to the lives of others.

Awareness

We can't do anything to understand or support menopausal women if we don't know anything about the menopause. Before thoughts of piles of dusty medical tomes and long, late nights in bafflement and resentment clouds the imagination, we don't need to be experts. The investment in time is minimal. There are easily accessible resources that won't be embarrassing to be seen reading in public. I'm fairly sure that no-one who reads this essay has ever actually seen a man reading a book about the menopause in public. How would you react if you saw such a thing? Would you shake their hand – or your head?

We should research early. If we postpone our awareness until we may need it, we'll already be lagging. The menopause doesn't arrive by recorded delivery, it's often a stealthy, incremental advance. It catches women out, too. Because popular culture depicts that they'll be drawing their pension by the time it arrives, they're often not ready either. There's not a critical path to it – we can find out first. Imagine that.

We should share our learning. As with many subjects we may research, validating what we discover, asking questions, seeking views, is all extremely helpful. It's suggested that it's not, therefore, an entirely lonely (and secret) pursuit. It could be that the person we share our learning with is the pre-menopausal or perimenopausal woman herself, which is equally fine.

We have to understand the range and scope of the menopause. In establishing that the experience is unique for every woman, as broad a perspective as possible is helpful. We may gain a deep awareness of our partner's encounter and assume that those with whom we interact at a similar stage at work are going through the very same, which is unlikely. If we're going to help, an open mind is essential. If we're not, then we really need to take a good look at ourself.

This is just preparation. If this opening aspect feels daunting, be assured it's the easy part.

Openness

If we've researched the menopause and engaged with others in ensuring our knowledge is broad and flexible, we've created the conditions to confidently interact in the scenarios mentioned earlier – at home, at work and in our relationships. That's not always easy when we're more accustomed to, and comfortable with, remaining on mute. But the knowledge we'll have amassed needs to be put to beneficial use.

We can be open reactively and proactively. The former is by far the easiest. That is, we'll be aware that the menopause is affecting behaviour or disposition, but it hasn't to date been raised. We're all not saying what needs to be said. Our role is to create the conditions for it to be articulated, in the form of space and time. Space being the physical environment and those present. Time being the removal of undue pressure, and a calm that builds trust. Whereas at present every woman would be generally right in thinking that raising the subject would generate a male response on a scale of bemusement to horror, the creation of a conducive situation may persuade her that an admission would be met with informed understanding.

Proactively is, as you may expect, much more difficult. Societally, we're a long way from a man being the one to raise the issue. As with offering congratulations on a pregnancy that's merely a little over-indulgence at the bakery, casually but confidently asking a spontaneously combusting woman "menopause is it, love?" is likely to invite a commensurate response. Unless we're medically qualified, and even if we are and aren't in a surgery or consulting room at the woman's request, we never raise it. In years to come, perhaps, this advice may change.

When the matter is surfaced and acknowledged, our ability to be open in talking about it will need to follow. This may entail surmounting a level of discomfort not yet attained. Most vitally, our role is to listen. We're irritatingly predisposed to dominance, drawing a situation into a rudimentary, often condescending explanation, and offering a fix. A menopausal woman doesn't need our advice, and certainly not our hastily-quacked remedy. We're there to absorb. The menopause represents a frontier of male maturity. Just in front of which is a bottomless ravine carefully disguised as expected behaviour.

Openness isn't necessarily easier in one of our three situations than the others. In each of a home in which ships pass silently, a work environment devoid of trust, a relationship characterised by introspection or the tentative steps of a first encounter, openness is challenged. It's not to say, either, that we might not be facing several simultaneously. We've assumed up to this point that it may just be a single occurrence. Our partner, sister, line manager and several of our team could all be experiencing the menopause simultaneously. It could be a whirlpool.

Responsiveness

We're now called on to do something about it. That doesn't mean staying out of the way, or simply staying out. Even if on the odd occasion a tactful low profile may be helpful. The situation – home, work or relationship – together with the pattern and seriousness of the symptoms will prompt the action needed. For the avoidance of doubt or on-rushing lack of commitment, there *will* be action needed.

We must remember, too, that we may be among the few aware of the situation. We don't wish to run ahead of our menopausal colleague across the open office ringing a bell in order to clear a safe path. We may have been trusted with a confidence and it absolutely has to remain as such, through our words and actions. In such instances there's only one chance on offer.

Principally driven by the complexity and unpredictability of the menopause, it will necessitate us broadening the limited palette of responses that were fitted as standard. Action comes in two forms – reactive and proactive. The reactive is simple – something's happening and we have to do something about it to stop or alleviate it. It's unlikely to be the former. We'll be working with it. We'll develop an understanding of each symptom and learn what we need to do. There will be times when we don't feel like it, where it's an occurrence too many. Yet imagine being the one experiencing it. Menopause is 24/7. For the avoidance of doubt that's all day, every day.

The proactive is far more difficult. How do we anticipate what's going to be needed when we're never sure what's going to happen? An entire plan based on all forty symptoms is beyond the scope of this essay, but several examples are given below for those more commonly experienced, set against the situation in which we're most likely to encounter them:

SYMPTOM	SITUATION	RESPONSE
Digestive problems	Home	A diet needs to be researched, planned and shared. It's likely to consist of more that's grown than manufactured. The vindaloo may have to be an occasional treat. Processed food, sugar and caffeine also negatively impact anxiety, too.
Hot flushes	Anywhere	When a hot flush hits, it's instantaneous. To be prepared, we need to choose cooler places – whether for a meeting or dinner out or vacation. Which means we might be in that same cooler place and need to remember to have our tank top to hand.
Anxiety	Anywhere	Simplify life – remove the clutter, physically and emotionally. Create conditions of calm. Visual interference will create mental interference. In a work environment, clear expectations, a manageable workload and an allowance for regular breaks are all helpful (they are for everyone, it's a pity that it still needs to be said).

SYMPTOM	SITUATION	RESPONSE
Memory loss	Anywhere	We have to manage our expectation of what will be recalled. We'll have to fill in the gaps. Saying "remember to fill the car up with petrol" is a guaranteed half mile walk with a jerry can. Have notebooks and pens handy and visible. Be the one to remember everything and ensure polite but ready prompts.
Difficulty concentrating	Work	Much depends on the nature of the role and opportunities within the physical environment to focus without disturbance. Allowances can be made, including working from home where possible.
Vaginal dryness	Relationship	This challenges a whole bucketload of masculinity. It's not about us, our failure to arouse. Pressure will exacerbate the situation. Lubricant is essential, and it has to be natural, organic and designed for women or it'll create further problems. Its application can be a shared aspect of intimacy. It needs to be readily available, not in the back of the wardrobe.

In considering the above, what seemed like an impossible task now appears practical and achievable. Those few suggestions are by no means exhaustive, either.

Togetherness

For those men in a relationship with a menopausal woman, there's a further contribution we can make. While men don't have a menopause, they're often having one vicariously. Which means unlike in passing interactions in a family, social or work environment, they're far closer to the symptoms and their consequences.

Symptoms require a response, and that response can be something we agree to partake in. If it means eating, drinking, behaving in particular ways, we both do it. The risk of developing osteoporosis, a reduction in bone density increasing the possibility of fracture, is exacerbated by menopause. Reducing alcohol intake is a key mitigation. For irresistibly social couples familiar with the odd hazy evening every weekend, this can have a direct impact on lifestyle. It's not a sparkling reason to ensure your partner drives you home while you sing *Bohemian Rhapsody* to yourself.

As symptoms are constant and unpredictable, togetherness is not something that can be switched on and off. It's a commitment. Full, undiluted and sincere. While we may wonder to ourselves as the novelty of the initial determination to beat the bugger wanes just how long the damn thing will go on for, the reality is that it's a journey not an event. We'll need several re-sets and re-appraisals, and the odd slippage in the new rules. It's not a tyranny. Remaining human – irrational, vulnerable, emotional – is not just to be expected, it's essential.

THE SECOND PHASE

Focus on the second phase of womanhood, when the menopause is finally over, is incredibly scant. Most literature on the menopause is locked in the sympathy/empathy vortex for the duration and concludes with the last cold towel. In reality, the menopause ends with neither a bang nor a whimper, it simply fades. Some symptoms fade quicker than others. There may be the odd reprise, just for old time's sake. When least expected, naturally.

The woman whose menopause has faded will be around 55 years old. That's still far enough from retirement to achieve remarkable things. Not the pensionable, safe-hobby, sensibly-shod geriatric depicted in most media. For men, there is much to learn. Just when, after four decades of painstaking trial-and-error reconnaissance we think we've understood women, they transform themselves and we have to recycle our copious notes and start over.

It's all about eggs, once again. Or, rather, their absence of them and the hormones that accompany them. The chemical disposition to caring, to putting others before themselves as mothers and partners that appeared innate is re-wired. Second phase women are likely to put themselves first. That certainly doesn't mean they don't care or aren't capable of caring – it's just that we're on notice.

Which is why organisations are damned fools for letting women slip away during menopause. It's a short-sighted convenience for them, born of ignorance: the difficult, inconsistent, unreliable and occasionally under-performing nuisance has walked, thankfully. She never used to be like that, it's a shame, but hey. It's not an exclusively male position, either. Even women whose menopause hasn't been as severe or have been fortunate that their support network has rallied to them can be of this view.

When the menopause is over, second phase women can be formidable. Capable, motivated and energised. All of which is great news for us if we're delighted for women to be more successful than us, a disaster if we're locked in a miserably patriarchal mindset. Which is probably why, given the tangle of agendas that defines an organisation, women are allowed to leave by women and men alike. They're a threat. 'The organisation' is itself a sum of its people. It doesn't get an objective say.

Second phase women can be far more capable of defining their relationships, too. Those men who opted to drop down the age scale to a pre-menopausal model so as not to have to face the prospect of being caring and responsive may never get to reap the benefit of a confident and liberated partner, sure of what she wants. It's just as possible that, if we haven't been there for her during the menopause, she'll look at us and decide it's not us she wants. We won't have changed, grown, matured, we'll just be an achier and grumpier version of who we once were. And she'd be right.

FROM HERE

We're out. The menopause is over. We knew what was to come, prepared ourselves, opened ourselves to the challenge, and responded. We were there for our family, colleagues and partner. We might permit ourselves a congratulatory smile as we contemplate the motivation and joy of the women in our life. We might also spare a thought for those who didn't take the opportunity to do likewise – and resolve that we'll ensure that our sons, brothers, friends and workmates awaken to the menopause and be the men within.

Reflections

Reflections

Reflections

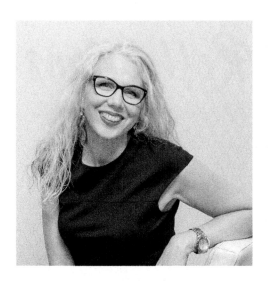

KATE USHER
UK

Kate is an experienced Menopause Coach and Change Strategist and specialist in gender equality. She works with women and organisations to create simple strategies that enable modern and supportive menopause conversations. This increases awareness of this life phase, its pivotal impact on equality across the workforce and representation in senior and executive positions.

She is an internationally published author. Her book 'Your Second Phase – reclaiming work and relationships during and after Menopause' was shortlisted for the Business Book of the Year Award 2021.

To discover more about Kate and the work she does, visit https://secondphase.co.uk

Chapter Six

POWER IN THE WORK PLACE

Firstly, I need to establish some facts or possibly ground rules. Each one of the authors in this book will gift you a way of being to manage your menopause journey, I strongly suggest you take them on board. Because as we all know menopause can be utterly shit, true for some it will be shitter than others but generally who would ask for this situation, right? Wrong!

You or the person you know, is travelling through a transition that only women get to experience. Our whole body is managing the withdrawal from both addictive and important chemicals, or as we know them hormones. For some of us this process of cold turkey is violent, at least that was my experience while others drift slowly in a serene and steady state. If I were to say that I am not envious of the latter I would be lying.

Even with this experience as my backdrop, I see the menopause as a wakeup call to establish healthy and supportive habits. Your body is telling you that you can no longer eat, drink and behave in a way that is unsupportive. You need to consider you, what is best for you in a holistic sense and what will make your heart sing. You are being coaxed towards opportunities to view this as a new beginning. In short, this is all about you.

Back to those facts. I live in the UK and as such the figures I will work to are those that are applicable here. Please feel free to amend them as per your own region/country.

- The average age of menopause is fifty-one
- Five per cent of women have their menopause before the age of forty-five and one per cent before the age of forty
- According to the NHS the average time that women will experience symptoms for is seven years (that's day and night for every one of those years, there is no day off)
- By 2025, twelve per cent of the world's population will be menopausal
- There are thirteen million menopausal women in the UK
- Twenty per cent of the UK working population are menopausal
- Twenty-five per cent of women consider leaving paid employment because of their menopausal symptoms
- Ten per cent of all women leave paid employment because of their menopausal symptoms

I work with women who are looking to maintain their hard fought for careers, and organisations who want to retain the incredible women who work for them. My focus is on creating a gender balanced workforce, increasing female representation at senior management and executive level. If we are to achieve it, we must incorporate menopause support and break the taboo that surrounds it. If we don't, more women will fall by the wayside at the final furlong. This is the stark and unpalatable truth.

It is time to take our collective head out of the sand and take action.

Repeatedly I speak to women who would rather knawe off their right arm than declare they are menopausal, even when they are having multiple hot flushes an hour, severe mood swings and/or crushing anxiety to name a few. Their colleagues are obviously aware that there is something going on, especially if they have had to deal with unexpected tears or shouting.

The issue that underpins this is that generally women and men are not aware of what the menopause is, what the symptoms are and how they might show up on a day-to-day basis. This is not surprising because we simply don't talk about it enough, this added to the fact that mind reading skills are not prevalent, means that without some form of declaration we go around thinking that Woman A or Woman B are being particularly unreasonable or unpredictable. This after all is a common slight aimed at women over the age of forty, so much so we rarely challenge it whether it be due to a widely held social myth, or by asking the woman in question what might be causing these changes, for fear of crossing some imaginary line.

The answer to this is for women to speak up and speak out, preferably with their right arm intact.

Why do we fear speaking out?

The easy answer is we don't want to be labelled as old. But that is too simplistic.

While menopause as a phrase was first coined by French doctor Charles Pierre-Louis de Gardanne in 1821, Aristotle has been quoted as referencing it and it has been discussed for centuries. Our grandmother's generation or at least the women who were born at the turn of twentieth century were the first to experience their menopause en masse. Prior to that only the lucky few lived long enough, menopause was a novelty that could be demeaned and dismissed as part of women's ageing experience. The issue for this generation was that their life expectancy was such that they died shortly after they became postmenopausal[1]. My own paternal grandmother was a prime example, she died aged fifty-two.

Life was hard for these women. Many were repeatedly pregnant, for many standards of living and nutrition were poor. Their generation had been robbed of many men due to the first world war, watched their sons follow a similar fate in the second world war, and struggled

---

1   ONS

through a devastating depression in between. In short, by the time they reached their late forties their bodies had endured much, and they looked like women would in their seventies and eighties today. This is not a criticism.

I cannot imagine how a woman would discuss vaginal atrophy with her husband or with her doctor who was undoubtedly male. Given that the NHS was not created until 1948 most women would not have had the financial means to access any form of medical support anyway.

Having said all of this, our grandmothers gave us an incredible gift which took great sacrifice from a relatively small number of women. One of whom was one of the most famous menopausal women of all, Emmeline Pankhurst. It was of course the right to vote. This generation also gained the right to divorce on the same grounds as men (Matrimonial causes act 1937).

Our mothers

Our mothers while entering the workforce, usually depending on social class and status, left when they got married and had children. For those who wished to continue working there was what was quaintly called the marriage bar, which is fairly self-explanatory. It meant that women were prevented from working once they were married (or widowed). The bar was removed slowly but was not removed fully until the 1970s. The knock-on effect of this was that women were not invested in in the workplace, they were not trained or offered jobs of worth because their time working was deemed temporary. For those that chose to focus on their career, they were often passed over as senior or jobs of worth were deemed as necessary for men to support their families, including their wives who were at home unable to work. The irony is not lost.

This has defined an approach to women in the workplace that still lurks in the shadows today. During the pandemic, the British government thanked women for all the work that they had done in the home, picking up the lion's share of housework, childcare and home schooling. The assumption was driven by an unspoken expectation of women as primary carers not career driven financially independent or primary household earners. This came at a price as women's wellbeing and mental health came under attack, as they tried to do all of this whilst maintaining their careers. This and other comments made at the time were rightly ridiculed and belittled for their sexist and outmoded message.

As is so often the case, changing perceptions about women's role in the workplace is more difficult than changing the law, which in itself is difficult enough. We are still fighting to gain equal opportunities and equal pay for equal work.

This generation without doubt fought their equality battles for equal pay (Equal Pay Act 1970) and demonstrated against cruise (nuclear) missiles at Greenham Common as well as the removal of the marriage bar and the right to have financial independence.

My mother states that menopause was not discussed, ever, not even amongst women.

There must have been knowing glances, but the mass contribution to effective management of the menopause appears to have been the cardigan. Beloved by the twinset and pearls set, enabling women to discreetly take it off and put it on repeatedly. Of course, this helped no other symptom than hot flushes. HRT made its first appearance to this generation but the understanding of the impact of taking hormones (taken from pregnant horse urine) was low. The first women taking it in the 1960s effectively acted as an ongoing clinical trial. Our understanding has developed considerably since that time, but there is too little investment and research in this area.

For our mothers, the societal taboo was so firmly in place that women were discouraged from discussing menopause amongst themselves, let alone with their husbands and partners or with their children. Us. There is no blame in this comment.

Then comes us

We are only two steps away from the first generation to experience the menopause en masse. In addition to this we are the first to gain an education, a career possibly alongside having children and to experience our menopause in the workplace.

Societally this is a new experience for everyone.

Women often lament that it isn't fair that this generation has to be the first. Again. While this might be true it is the way it is. We can either break the taboo or live with it and all the limitations that it brings. Most women choose to smash it with whatever metaphorical weapon they need. Anger is a menopausal symptom and I often wonder if it is nature's way of firing us to drive change.

I frequently ask in workshops for a show of hands (men and women), whether they had heard menopause discussed openly at home when they were growing up? Generally, there is a maximum of two and more commonly, zero. We all arrive at menopause unaware and uninformed. The only exception to this is popular myths, and when I say popular, I mean we all know them. I have yet to meet a woman who likes them.

Popular menopause myths

These are not only generated by history and a male medicalised view, but also the media from the 1960s to 1990s. Every single view we had of women over the age of forty was negative, we were depicted as past our prime, busy bodies and difficult. We fell into two camps either matronly or trying too hard to prove we were still attractive. None of these are good role models for us as women as we approach these years, nor are they positive stereotypes to subconsciously call on when the word menopause is uttered.

Most of us will remember the horror of the hairdresser's drying pods where older women sat lined up against the wall, waiting with curlers tightly clipped for their hair to dry. They looked more like victims of an alien invasion. These women linger in our subconscious, house coats on (a cross between a large apron and a lab jacket), bodies devastated by multiple pregnancies and poor dental hygiene. The issue here is that these are the images we drag forth once menopause is mentioned. There is a toxic mix of conscious, subconscious and confirmation bias that wraps itself like a straitjacket around the word, the myth, the experience we call menopause.

We all, women and men experience bias, it is part of the human condition. It is our brain's way of conserving energy. We fill gaps with assumptions learnt while growing up e.g., when X happens that means Y, or when A occurs, I do B and then C. This is so that we don't have to think our way through every single thought and experience. It would be exhausting. The interesting thing however is that our bias is not hard wired, we can absolutely change our opinion and beliefs about anything whether it be sexism, racism or homophobia to name a few. The caveat here is that it takes time and consistent effort. After all, they were not established and then reinforced in a moment. Here is the fantastic thing about it, identifying unhelpful or outmoded bias signals an opportunity. Once you are aware of it you can change it. So instead of feeling seriously uncomfortable about thinking something and stuffing it back down into the dark recesses of your mind, step into your discomfort, unpack it, recognise where it came from and begin the process of changing your thinking.

Women of menopausal age today are stylish, modern and self-defined. Very few line up to be the homogenised or stereotyped woman many of us visualise when the word menopause is mentioned. We are part of a generation that rebelled against the establishment, the grey, brown dourness of the 1970s and a bleak employment outlook. We became punks and new romantics, pink mohawks, mohair jumpers and safety pins or wedges, big perms, frilly shirts and lots of makeup for both women and men. We felt like we could change the world. Not fit into it.

So why three or four decades on are we fighting to break free of societal limitations again? We are not our mothers or our grandmothers the lives we have lived to this point are dramatically different. Even if we chose not to take them, the opportunities we have been offered are vastly different. We have had to write our own story, define our own path. It really is time to break the stereotypes, dig in, find that rebel that burned inside you. There is a lot to fight for.

IMPACT

What is the impact of not changing our perceptions? Why should we bother? Surely by raising the issues around menopause in the workplace we are in fact limiting our progression, defining ourselves as trouble and ultimately making ourselves unemployable?

I would like to remind you that women rarely get anything gifted to them unless they aggravate the status quo. Before the term 'Disrupters' dances across your consciousness, I pulled back from using it as it feels kitsch and flippant in this context. Our right to vote, removal of the marriage bar, equal pay for equal work, maternity leave and parental leave even the #MeToo movement, 'Reclaim the night' and #EverydaySexism are all examples of this. By being prepared to question and aggravate how things are done, we have established changes in the law or new levels of social consciousness that are for many, taken for granted. We should always question 'the way it's always been' because rarely is that good for women.

We do not make ourselves unemployable, we make ourselves and the generations of women behind us more employable. We are highlighting our skills, value and contribution. We are drawing attention to what we do and why losing that is not only costly on many levels it removes the path for future generations to progress along. Last and by no means least we are highlighting our contribution to the commercial success of the organisation - if the moral position is not strong enough - quite frankly any employer that takes this position should see swathes of employees whether they are female or male getting their CVs together – then the financial argument is. The cost of replacing some of the most talented and knowledgeable members of staff is extremely high.

Impact on women

Firstly, if women think that the mere mention of menopause will invoke derisory comments from colleagues or managers, or that they will be the butt of numerous derogatory, ageist and sexist jokes, they will endeavour to push on through no matter how hard it is. This is not an exaggeration the TUC, a British trade union, found in their 2016 survey that 58.5 per cent of the respondents witnessed menopause being treated as a joke. If women feel that being identified as menopausal will impact both their current and long-term job prospects, they will remain silent. In the report undertaken by the Fawcett Society for Standard Chartered Bank and the Financial Services Skills Commission (2021) they found that only twenty-two per cent of women and trans men declared their menopause status, this is catastrophic for an industry where one in ten of those who work within it, are menopausal. This is without doubt within the sphere of psychological and elemental safety. In addition to this the Equalities act (2010) protects people against such behaviour on the grounds of age, sex and depending on severity of symptoms, disability.

Health

Firstly, women push themselves too far in an attempt to drift swan like through the menopause. If this is you then the damage you are doing to your physical, mental and emotional wellbeing is considerable. Your body is changing and you can no longer take it for granted. Stress, sleep deprivation and weight gain are a three-pronged attack, which is common at this time in life. They have wide reaching health implications. The top four are:

Heart disease – very much a female issue post menopause.

Diabetes – our propensity to weight gain can very easily get out of hand.

Alzheimer – stress and inflammation are the focus of recent research into why women outnumber men 2:1 when it comes to this disease.

Osteoporosis – A silent killer and one which we don't tend to consider until it is making its impact known on our mobility.

Struggling through, fighting to keep our head above water when realistically we feel like we are drowning, drives a sense of isolation. This is compounded when we feel unable to seek help or support or confide in a colleague. The darkness and desperation that inveigles its way into our consciousness at this point, is scary and should be taken notice of. There is always a way to switch the light on but the longer we leave it the more difficult it is to find the light switch.

The sense of loneliness is something women always talk about, and for me even as I write this it always brings me to tears to hear it, because I walked this path and know how unnecessary this anguish is.

Is it any wonder that women choose to scale back their career or worst of all leave paid employment altogether, rather than declare?

Reputation

You have worked bloody hard for at least two decades to get the career you have now. You have had to deal with the glass ceiling, glass walls and the greasy pole to achieve it. You have worked extraordinary hours, managed upwards and downwards. If you have had children, you will have watched as others were promoted due to evening networking events or excessive international travel, while you elected to get home to collect your child/children from nursery or school. To be around to see their first steps, hear their first words and weep at the annual nativity play, whether they were a donkey or one of the highly coveted lead roles. These moments are truly irreplaceable, whether you are the parent or the child who knows you are out there supporting and loving them.

You have driven yourself hard to regain a modicum of lost ground and felt that you were back where you needed to be, to be in with a shout for promotion. Then your menopause happened.

Maybe there were imperceptible changes that slowly developed until one day you forgot something or burst into tears about an issue you would previously have shrugged off. Perhaps you shouted at someone for a comment that would not have registered on your radar but is now a major afront. These are effectively the claxon that sounds as your hormones dip below a point that your body can smooth over.

Suddenly you can find yourself in a place that you are completely unprepared for. The unpredictability of menopause can feel damaging to your professional reputation and authority. Not knowing which version of yourself will turn up in any given moment can be devastating to your confidence. This is a downward spiral that only picks up speed.

Managing your changing self requires conscious action.

Finance

For some reason women don't feel comfortable talking about money. One woman asked me to take out the section on money in my book 'Your Second Phase.' This is ludicrous, in my opinion we need to talk about money a whole lot more, especially as so many women are now the sole or principal earners in their household. We are go-getters in the office and housewives with our bank accounts. Ladies if you are in the workplace earning your own money, learn how to manage it in a way that is not akin to the little woman and her housekeeping money. We are taught that money is a male responsibility that it has a male energy about it. Bollocks. It doesn't feel so male when you can't pay your bills or feed yourself or your children. It is time to take that money bull by the horns and tame it. Make that money that you worked so hard for, now work hard for you. Money is simply an enabler that we need, to pay for things to help us live. Yes, the more you have the more luxuriant those things are, but let's not get hung up on the moral argument around money. You worked for it. You earnt it. You look after it.

One quick word on equal pay … we work hard for our money and deserve the success that it brings. We are sadly a long way off gaining true salary parity with men. In 2021 the Fawcett Society announced that Equal Pay Day was 18th November, in 2021 it was 20th November. This is the date from which women effectively work for free, whereas men continue to be paid for the remainder of the year. The imbalance exists for CEOs as it does for admin assistants. No one is exempt.

The specific financial issue for women during menopause is that many choose, where there is no workplace support, to scale back their careers while they manage their symptoms, or in extreme cases choose to leave paid employment altogether. Believe me I understand. Within six months of my menopause kicking in, it took everything I had to get my then little children to school in the morning.

By scaling back your career you are effectively blocking your progress at least for the foreseeable future. The effort required to crank up your career again later down the line is considerable, realistically you may not get the opportunity to achieve the levels you might previously have sought.

This will of course impact your current and future salary. It will in turn impact your potential pension. This is a big decision, with far reaching implications.

If you choose to leave employment altogether this is in effect the nuclear option. Yours and potentially your family's financial wellbeing is at stake, in both the short and long term for the reasons I have highlighted above.

Before you choose either option, I ask for you to think this through with a clear mind, considering all the ramifications. I will in the 'Way Forward' section discuss the steps you can take to help yourself.

Impact on organisations

In a recent report from the Fawcett Society working with Standard Chartered Bank and the Financial Services Skills Commission, it stated that fifty per cent of those surveyed chose not to take on extra responsibilities, that is, step back from their promotion opportunities.

As per the facts at the beginning of this chapter twenty-five per cent of women consider leaving employment due to their menopausal symptoms. Ten per cent do, taking with them decades of knowledge, awareness, experience and capability. For many this is more about a lack of awareness in the wider workforce that drives a hostile workplace. This underpinned by the lack of a meaningful strategy to support women through this phase in life. In figures just released by the British government only twenty five per cent of organisations have a menopause policy or guidelines. This places the remaining seventy five per cent in a vulnerable position especially as the number of tribunal cases citing menopause in 2021 is predicted to quadruple the number reported in 2018.

There is much at stake.

Loss of talent

At a time when there is a dearth of talent, it is nonsensical to open the door to losing some of your most brilliant and experienced employees. Women at this time in their career are just as men in their ascendency. They have decades of industry, organisation and function experience. They understand how to get things done, who to speak with and how to achieve excellence in a climate that desperately needs those skills.

All of this is difficult to quantify as far as costs are concerned however the loss of women at this point means the existing investment that they represent in working hours, training and development, is instantly lost. The interconnected nature of your workforce means that the role they played in achieving results both formal and informal is lost as well.

Women want to see other women in senior management positions, if women are either stepping back or leaving at a critical point in their career, other women will interpret this rightly or wrongly as an indicator that they are not valued and choose an employer that offers visible and open support.

Recruitment

Women of all ages seek to see each other. If they are underrepresented no amount of spin will hide the lack of recognition of female excellence. The term 'If you can't see it, you can't be it,' is at play here. Women want to see an established pathway to seniority no matter how lightly trodden. In a recent Cranfield University report, sponsored by Ernst & Young a global professional services company, it highlighted that only 13.2 per cent of the FTSE 100 executive directors are female whereas it was a meagre 11.3 per cent in the FTSE 250.

On this point we must not let ourselves get distracted by the voluntary thirty-three per cent (Davis Report 2015) quota for female non-executive directors (NEDs). NEDs do not influence the day to day running of an organisation nor do they define or nurture the culture. They are there in an advisory capacity and to create a check point as and when is necessary. In addition to this NEDs tend to have a portfolio of boards that they sit on. Which could mean that the same woman is counted a maximum of six times. Suddenly the picture looks even less diverse. This being said, the work done by the Davis Report and the Hampton-Alexander Report has been invaluable in raising the recognition of a lack of female representation at a senior level. The reality is however that some organisations fulfil the board quota then have a male only executive team that drives the organisation underneath it, which to all intent and purposes is out of view. These days however a little persistent searching easily reveals a diverse or non-diverse executive and senior management team.

If organisations want to recruit the best talent available, visibility matters, it influences people's decision to apply for roles. This of course means excellent candidates don't even press send, reducing the potential talent pool. Let's be clear this is not just young people but those of all ages and seniority.

Networks

Women are great networkers, but because traditional networking has been based around an extension of the gentleman's club, it has subliminally excluded them by it being based around boozy after work events, when women need to get home to their family, or corporate entertainment which is often based around male dominated sports such as golf, football and rugby, many women have sought to create their own network groups. They are environments where women can talk about the things that matter to them and enable them to reach their ambitions amongst female allies and mentors.

There are two issues here. Firstly, women are excluded from influential relationship building and deal making by this male centric approach to networking. This situation reinforces the male advantage and female disadvantage. Secondly, which is where poor support for menopause has an impact, women talk about their employers and either recommend them to each other or seek to leverage their relationships, to move elsewhere. Negative perceptions and female talent travel fast.

Reputation and brand value

Every organisation wants to be an employer of choice, they want their employees, peers, suppliers and customers proud to be associated with them.

Marks & Spencer and John Lewis, major high street brands in England both loved and cherished by the middle classes, recognise the importance of openly talking about how they support their female staff through the menopause. Internally it is the right thing to do, as both have a high percentage of female staff who hold considerable knowledge and experience, in a highly competitive retail market. Outwardly, it positively reinforces the relationship with both brand's customers. Women of menopausal age are highly influential on the high street, with higher levels of disposable income than their younger counterparts. It is an easy win; women of menopausal age want to see their counterparts respected and supported throughout this transition. For any organisation, a tribunal or even internal rumours (remember those networks?), would be extremely damaging to both their brand and their reputation. Did I say it's a highly competitive market?!

Got the picture?

Historically we thought of menopause as a 'woman's issue' that the impact is to be born solely by women. I hope by now that there is a dawning realisation that this is a woman, man, organisation and societal issue and one that can no longer be ignored.

From a business perspective the reticence to enter this space must be managed and resolved. Women are an incredible force are being allowed through inaction to either step into the shadows or walk out the door. The global nature of business requires the contribution that women make. McKinsey reported that those organisations with a gender diverse senior management team, outperformed those who did not by twenty-five per cent. Menopause support is a cornerstone in enabling women to reach those senior roles. The benefits are clear and easy to attain.

WAY FORWARD

After the storm comes the sun.

For you as a woman

I am here to tell you that menopause whilst utterly shit, at times is an opportunity. It is without doubt a power phase in our lives. Unfortunately, we have been told over centuries that it and all its shitty symptoms are the end of all that is good in our lives. Unsurprisingly we don't want to think about it, talk about it or experience it. Tough shit lady, we all have to.

Whilst we collectively insist on wallowing in our own pool of self-pity and only speaking in hushed and dour tones about menopause, we invite unscrupulous members of our community both male and female to dismiss us.

Where is the punk that once roared at the establishment or the new romantic that changed the face of youth music and fashion or the rave goer that broke all the laws to be part of an irrepressible youth culture? All these groups valued equality, blurred the lines of gender, stuck two fingers up to racism and accepted each other for what they were. May I suggest she is still in there, swearing and drinking snake bites, Diamond Whites or for the more avant garde rum and cokes.

If you are to break the unspoken yet expected slide into anonymity, you will need the fire of her to drive you through the dark times and to actualise the opportunity that menopause represents.

Decisions, decisions

Menopause is both an end and a beginning. You are passing from the first to the second phase of your womanhood. Unlike the first, you arrive at this second phase educated, able and experienced. Which means emancipation is yours for the taking.

You are free to choose what happens next. As your hormone levels change and return to a prepubescent steady state you are moving from the back of the queue, as far as needs are concerned, to the front. This is where you will remain for the rest of your life.

With this in mind, what do you want for yourself?

If you were to roll forward five or ten years, where do you want to be, what do you want to be doing and who do you want to be doing it with?

These are big questions that deserve the time to be thought through. They are even more impactful if you recognise that you really do have the opportunity to refocus your life and ambitions in whichever direction you choose.

As far as work is concerned, if you are of average perimenopausal age, you have enough time – twenty years – for a second career. It's a long way off retirement.

Do you have ambitions for the 'C' Suite, do you want a portfolio career, or have a burning idea that the previously dormant entrepreneur inside you, is desperate to take to market? Now is the time to focus on it. Remember there is much at stake, not least your financial wellbeing, both now and in the future. You really are worth the time it takes to think this through.

This knowledge will also drive your approach at work. Whatever you choose for yourself, it is important that decisions are not based on the current status quo. If you are having a crap time and your symptoms are drowning the person inside, now is the time to take action, for yourself. This book is filled with opportunities for action, not all of them will resonate with you and your unique experience. But each chapter will gift you something whether that be a new perspective, guidance or support. Take it.

One of the most disempowering features of our current approach to menopause is the lack of options we provide for ourselves. If you need additional support, take it, whether it be focussing on your diet, lifestyle or the way you think about yourself. Your body is absolutely calling for change.

It is not an underestimation to say that the changes and decisions that you make now, form the foundation for your future. As you move up the queue, put you first.

Speaking up and speaking out

You are not alone in feeling unsure about this step, however for all the reasons previously stated, if your symptoms are showing up in a way that affects how you work or interact with others, it really is time to take control of what happens next.

Speaking out does two things, firstly it enables you to define the narrative around you and your symptoms, removing the opportunity for rumour or malicious comments. Secondly, it gives you the opportunity to access the support you need, to keep your career on track or moving in the direction you wish it to.

You and your symptoms

The first step is to be clear about what your symptoms are. Quite literally make a list. Without this information you are working in the dark. It is important to state that this is not an opportunity to rake over past misdemeanours or events and ramp up the anxiety over what you could have or should have done. Neither is it the time to ignore certain symptoms so that you don't have to admit their impact. This is quite literally a cold hard list of facts.

Once this is complete identify how and when they show up. Many symptoms can be better or worse at certain times of day, whether that be due to fatigue, sleep, diet or hydration, while others seem to be fairly consistent.

Which brings us to the next category which is impact. Some symptoms while annoying will have very little impact, yet for others it will be profound. This process will begin to isolate those symptoms that are most troublesome from the rest of the pack.

It is important to reiterate here that each woman's experience is unique to her. Do not belittle yourself for not being able to cope, your menopause is unique to you. This route will rob you of the ability to take positive action and will take you down the disempowered rabbit hole.

This brings us to the last category, what support do you need to be able to continue with your chosen career? Would it be flexible working hours, cool or calm workplace spaces, breathable workwear, ready access to cold drinking water or the ability to switch the video off during the endless online meetings? These are just a few of the common adjustments women ask for to help them through this phase in life. The important thing is to think about which of your symptoms are most impactful and what would help you manage them better within the working environment.

I often advise women to rank their symptoms and the requested support/adjustments:

1 = Essential

2 = Nice to have

3 = Occasionally as and when needed

This way, you can see at a glance what you really need to ask for.

Policies and guidelines

What does your organisation have in place already? Twenty-five percent of UK businesses now have one or other in place. Obviously, that means that seventy-five per cent don't. If you find yourself working amongst the majority, think laterally: Do they have a strong wellbeing ethic? Have they supported other health and wellbeing initiatives before? A good example would be mental health. If the answer is yes, then you can follow an established process in raising issues.

If your organisation is one of the twenty-five per cent, take a look at what the policy or guidelines advise you to do by way of speaking to someone, there may be a preference for you to speak to HR or your manager. In addition to this, what adjustments do they offer and lastly do you need confirmation from your GP that you are menopausal, to access them?

Precedent:

What is the precedent in your team, department or organisation? What have other women experienced? How have they accessed support or adjustments and how have they maintained or adjusted them as time has gone on? Seek other women out that might be at some stage in their menopause journey, meet for a coffee whether it be face to face or virtual and basically get the gossip.

If no self-help group already exists, then start one. They cost nothing to form and are extremely supportive for women at this stage of life – whatever age they are.

The meeting:

First, you need to tell your manager or HR person that you would like to have a meeting and state that it's about menopause. It is important to tell them, so they can prepare as well. They need to ensure that they understand what can be offered by way of adjustment or support. You don't want to go through all this and then find that you have to do it all over again, because they are unsure how to proceed.

When thinking about this meeting, make sure it is at a time that suits you. If you are better in the morning or the afternoon, ensure you book the meeting within your preferred hours. Choose a place if you are meeting face to face where you will feel comfortable. If you have hot flushes, don't choose the corner meeting room that gets really hot due to solar gain, no matter how good the view is. The important thing is to control what you can, remember you are driving this.

Open the meeting with your intention which is to discuss and create a plan of support and adjustment to enable you to continue with your career. Remember this is a business negotiation, you are defining your working arrangements for the next few months at least, if not years.

Lastly make notes and give the other party a copy. If they make notes, ensure you get a copy of theirs too. Arrange a date and time for a review meeting with the understanding that this will need to be revisited periodically.

Remember, you are in control of the next phase of your career. Planning and preparation will ensure this conversation goes smoothly and successfully.

For organisations

Many organisations are starting to recognise the importance of supporting women through this phase in life. There are of course business reasons including the retention of some of their most brilliant employees, but for many they see it as a demonstration of care for the people who work for them. It is quite simply the right thing to do.

Awareness:

Change always begins with awareness. Menopause is one of those subjects that has been hidden away for so long that most of us only know it via myth and media misrepresentation. Sadly, this underpins bias. This spells trouble for any employer, as left unchecked it is a breeding ground for 'banter' and inappropriate and derogatory comments. Sometimes opening the door to issues that need not occur.

To address this, awareness must be for everyone. No exceptions.

Managers need to be trained in how to support their staff through this inevitable phase in life, it is unreasonable to expect them to seamlessly absorb this. The discomfort around menopause far exceeds that of the classic conversation around personal hygiene. Those who act as Sponsors and Mentors need to be aware of what menopause is and its impact. Without this unconscious bias can impact women's progression.

Awareness is not a once and done activity, it needs to be part of the onboarding process and annual compliance, that way it doesn't become a box ticking exercise that won't stand up to scrutiny.

Policies and guidelines

If you don't have either a menopause policy or guideline, then now is as good a time as any to get started. There are numerous consultants out there who can help you, including me of course. The advantage of going to market now with your new initiative, is that you can monopolise the media and PR airways, and most importantly, retain some of your most experienced staff and attract new employees.

A first step is to define what support you can realistically offer. SMEs are not in the same position as global corporates or even national brands, but there are still things that the smallest company can do. Cold water, desk fans, calm spaces, free sanitary ware in the loo and time off to see medical professionals, costs virtually nothing and can be done today. The larger the organisation the bigger the workforce and the associated budget for meaningful and flexible adjustments.

The biggest step is an openness to awareness, acceptance and support.

FINAL THOUGHTS

To conclude, menopause in the workplace is not a 'women's issue,' it is everyone's issue. Awareness across the organisation enables a foundation of understanding and empathy that is new to the working environment. Those in positions of power and influence need specialised and specific training to ensure that they can act without bias and intervene should they see negative or demeaning 'banter' or acts occurring.

There is much at stake for organisations. They wish to attract and retain the most experienced, knowledgeable and valuable people. Effective and flexible menopause support is a key enabler for this. The cost of negative and conversely the potential for positive PR around menopause, will drive women either towards or away from their metaphorical doors.

For women there is much to play for. They are the first generation to experience their menopause en masse in the workplace and as such it is tough to break through the historic bias around this phase in life. But we must, to retain our careers, salaries, pensions and wellbeing.

We need to educate ourselves and be prepared to step forward and ask for help, no matter how uncomfortable or difficult that is. If we do not declare the situation and push for appropriate and meaningful support, we effectively lose our right to complain, and for some, we jeopardise our careers.

We are more educated, experienced and knowledgeable than we have ever been. This partnered with a change in focus means we are a force to be reckoned with. We can only step into the power of this phase if we come out of the shadows and feel our full strength inside our skin, no matter how sweaty, itchy or dry it is.

We can, we must, and in the long run we will be pleased we did.

Reflections

Reflections

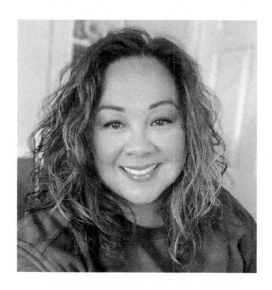

LAARNI MULVEY
USA

Filipino American Women's Strength Advocate, Mind Strength Coach, Author, Speaker, and Powerlifter, Laarni Mulvey, is the Founder of Strong and Mighty Company and the Global Standing in Strength Movement.

Her mission is to educate the world on the views of women and champion them to know they are stronger than they think they are.

She nurtures women to build a powerful legacy for themselves and future generations by providing resources to all realms of Strength.

Known as 'The Power Lady' she encourages and leads women to honour themselves through her message of Strength.

www.laarnimulvey.com

Chapter Seven

STRONG AND HAPPY

My period came when I was thirteen. I went to the bathroom and there was blood in my underwear. I literally tried to ignore it and thought 'No, this isn't it, is it?' which resulted in me changing my underwear about five times that day. The talk about having my period with my mother or my sister was something we never really talked about. My mum realised something was going on when I was going to the bathroom a lot. She came into my room and caught me hiding my underwear under a pile of clothes in my closet because I did not want to accept the idea of having my period or that I was becoming a woman. I figured if I continued to ignore the blood-stained underwear, then it did not happen. I didn't realise then that I was probably ashamed and even afraid.

My mum asked me in her Filipino accent "Did you get your period?"

With an embarrassing shrug, I said, "I guess."

She introduced me to using a maxi pad and said, "Put this in your underwear."

These were the late eighties and the style of maxi pad was far from the 'invisible with wings' panty liners we have today. They were about an inch thick and stiff as a board which left me feeling like a witch riding a broom. Looking back, I guess junior high sex ed class was the only real preparation for my period. My mum shared the news with the rest of the family, which was so embarrassing, but I assumed it was considered a proud moment to share that the family's little girl has become a 'woman.' The thought of having a period did not scare me. It was more the idea of a period being something socially embarrassing because I would stain my pants or leave a spot on the chair I was sitting on that time, I didn't think too much about then, but now, why is the first period considered that you are becoming a woman? Whoever said having a menstrual cycle is a blessing, never had the experiences that goes along with having a period.

Losing my virginity at fifteen, whilst dating someone in high school I thought I'd gotten pregnant. I find it amusing that I was not worried about getting some sexually transmitted disease but getting pregnant, becoming a teenage mum was a fear. The thoughts running through my mind included having to tell my family I was pregnant and seeing their reaction of disappointment. As I think back, my teenage years were a mess and filled with teenage angst, but I was looking for some kind of acknowledgment. Whether it be good or bad acknowledgment. Teenage pregnancy seemed right in the middle. I saw teenage pregnancy in high school as more of a curiosity to see what my parents would say and do.

I knew being a teenage mum meant my future would be over. No career, no life because I would be tied to a kid until they were eighteen. I continued to have sex anyway, protected of course, and I lived with the mindset of 'if I get pregnant, I get pregnant.' Whenever I did have a scare, I prayed hard to get my period. The first time in my life, I was thankful for the late arrivals of my period and prayed to God to give me my next period. I knew then, I feared having children over experiencing burning urination from a sexually transmitted disease.

SUPPOSED TO BE

Some people may consider my life path to be non-traditional. My life started in the Philippines, then I became an immigrant in the US at the age of five. America was the land of the free and full of opportunities. Living in America was going to be a fresh adventure handed to the five-year-old me, but it was not the case. Embracing the freedom of opportunities does not come easy when the box of conformity is handed to you at such an early age. There was an expectation for being a Filipina. I was supposed to be a docile, quiet Asian woman and live the inevitable mould of living by other people's standards and expectations. Whilst never openly instructed to do so, social pressures were forming this identity. It was an unspoken standard for me to be a nurse along with being a mother. My native culture was deeply programmed into me, and I love being Filipino.

Growing up as a Filipina in America added societal expectations upon me. The relationships and experiences I went through began to dictate my feelings about having children. At that time, it was stressed upon me that the only way to be accepted as a woman was to get married and have kids. Deep inside I felt, being a mother was the only way I would feel loved and to have a purpose. I really thought I wanted to have children because having children was going to save me and give me my purpose and my identity. I was so wrong in what my initial purpose and vision of my life was going to be. I wanted more than what I was supposed to be.

TEN YEARS GONE

In my twenties, I had no idea what I wanted to do with my life. I lived my life like any other twenty-something and enjoyed the club scene, drinking, partying, hanging out with my girlfriends, and men. Oh, the men!

In my professional career, I made the decision to do something that included being in athletics. The path to that decision started when I began junior college trying out new things and different classes. Even then, I really was not fully sure working in athletics was really what I wanted to do as a career. My sheltered upbringing made me want to work in athletics because it was when I felt most like my true self when lost in movement, fitness, and exercise. I knew eventually I wanted to be involved in athletics somehow.

Coming from a predominantly medically educated happy family, I compromised and combined my love for athletics and sports to pursue Athletic Training and Sports Medicine. What some people do not realise about Athletic Training is that the time demand is great. As a young single person in my mid-twenties or even in a serious romantic relationship, it was a perfect profession for me. When I entered the Athletic Training program, I was the oldest in the program which didn't bother me at all. I was able to hang with the younger students and I had my life outside of school. There were a few times I went to class hungover or still with the makeup I had on from the night before, which built more bridges than it burnt. Partying never stopped me from putting in my time into building my career. One day in the library, I was sitting next to my classmate. He had asked me if I was on Facebook. I said, 'What's that?' He asked me the sign-up questions, and then he said, 'Welcome to Facebook.' Remember, I was the oldest in the Athletic Training program. So, my response is similar now when someone says they don't have any social media and I have to explain what it is. After that, life got entertaining. What I started to see on social media was my friends having relationships, shared experiences, and building their families and their lives. Ten years of my life passed, and I was still not in a committed relationship or wanting to have children. At that time, I questioned the pressure on me to HAVE a husband and to HAVE children.

CAREER-DRIVEN

Once I graduated from being an undergrad, another four years of my life had passed, and I was still concentrating on my career. I was about to exit my twenties and my thirties were even closer on the horizon. Finding the right job to start my career was exciting and became my main focus. There was the judgment from people who did not understand why I was still single, especially when people would ask my age and I said thirty-two. After asking my age, and the initial shock wore off because I still looked like I was in my early twenties, this is the order of questions that would usually get asked and it would go in this order.

- Why are you still single? You are too pretty to be single.
- Don't you want to get married and settle down?
- When are you getting married so you can have a few kids?
- Do you like men?

The generality of the question of 'Why I wasn't married and why I was still childless' was always coming up from others.

I also wanted a career and not a job. Some people found it wrong and judged me for being a career-driven woman because when was I going to have time for a relationship. They would sometimes comment "Time is ticking…what are you waiting for?"

People started making assumptions about me. I was amused by the assumptions and the judgments pressured on the reasons why I should be in a relationship. Occasionally, the pressure to fulfill the mold of motherhood did get to me. Though I did not focus on having children, I did want a romantic relationship.

At the peak of my Athletic Training career, I would be at work sixty plus hours a week, more than twelve hours a day including the weekends. By that time, social media was showing everyone I knew getting married, having their kids, buying homes, and living their lives and I was working my butt off. I fell into the comparison trap, and I questioned what I had. When was I going to have a life like the other people I was seeing and when was it going to happen for me? I started to question where my life was going, and if and when was I going to meet the man of my dreams and start our lives together? Envy began to set in because I saw others living their lives and looking so happy. What I knew at that point was that to be happy, I was supposed to be building a family. I was wondering when my chance of *that kind of life* was going to happen. I was happy with my budding career, and I had to remind myself that I made the choice to go to school so I could have a career and not a job.

I also knew early on in my career I was going to focus on being an Athletic Trainer and work my way up to be in pro sports or to be an Athletic Trainer in the Olympics. I got into the profession not only because I loved being surrounded by athletes and sports, but it was going to be the closest I could get to being considered an athlete. Athlete by association. The Athletic Training profession demanded a lot of time away from home and a lot of time in the office. I loved being needed by my athletes, and it gave me the acknowledgment I sought when I was younger. I considered my athletes my kids even though they were adults. I experienced some kind of motherhood in that sense while taking care of my athletes.

The way my career was going, my future looked impressive. I was getting paid a good salary, lived on my own in my apartment with no roommates, and my little space had additional room available just in case there was an 'accidental' addition. Compared to the people I knew, I was one of the ones who was still dating and doing the single life, collecting stories from the bars and clubs. Besides the party stories, there were always new stories of traveling with my team, sports medicine injuries, life with my athletes, and the other fun reckless things that I was doing in my life.

I don't regret any of those stories by the way. I was happy.

Sometimes I do reminisce about those stories and laugh but those were my early life lessons and there are some things I know I will never do again...well maybe not.

The happy life didn't erase the pressures attached to the usual questions about being single. Those pressures weighed heavily on my mind and influenced future decisions. I rolled my eyes a lot when those questions were asked because it was tiresome and really no one's business. I decided the answer I would give to those questions was going to be lackadaisical and not put pressure on the idea. If I were going to have a family, get married, it was going to happen if and when it would happen. If it didn't happen, then it didn't happen. I was really set on that kind of no-pressure answer. Some people were cool with the answer and some people told me I was missing out on the best part of life. Until I reached that point, I was going to continue living my life so I could build the vision I saw for myself.

As my thirties began, the foundation of my life was becoming strongly rooted. I started to know what I wanted in my life, and I was beginning to have the confidence to choose my own path. It was a second turning point in my confidence. It became apparent to me in my mid-thirties what my choice of kids, relationships, and other adult things would be.

CALL ME SELFISH

My *'if and when'* answer about having kids as I reached my upper thirties marked me as selfish woman. Selfish because I was not focusing on having a relationship and because I was not focusing on having kids. I chose to be more focused on my career, and on the activities that I was going to do next and experiencing life's opportunities. To be seen as selfish was surprising, but something I had come to expect. So, if being too busy having fun, laughing, and living life was selfish, then so be it. I knew being a mother and a wife would not define me and would not be the only things to make me happy and whole.

When I started looking into getting into a meaningful relationship, I took a long hard look at my stance on having kids. How high was the priority of having kids on my relationship list? If I met someone who was one hundred per cent dating to have kids, those relationships did not work out. If it happened that I would get pregnant then I would have made it work, but it was not a priority.

I did not, and still don't believe my way of thinking is wrong. Yes, I go back and forth about absolutely wanting to be a mother and not being bothered either way, as I believe I would have been unhappy being a mum and I would have been a mother to please other people. I am not saying mothers are unhappy, and I commend mothers for their commitment. For me though, I made the decision for myself to be happy and take advantage of all the opportunities life brings me until life decides to make me a mother. Let me clarify, I love some other people's kids and I do not hate kids, it's just they are not a huge priority in my life. I'll happily babysit and entertain kids to keep them busy, but they are not something I focus on having in my life. Making these choices doesn't make me a selfish or irresponsible person, it just means I am choosing my life based on who I am, not who others want me to be to validate their own choices.

THE 'CHANGE'

As I said at the beginning of chapter, for me having periods was the absolute worst because back then we did not have period panties like we have now in 2022. We would need to wear heavy-duty pads, tampons, black pants, long skirts, or anything that was period-proof, that is, anything that wouldn't allow or show the leaks of heavy bleeding. We would need to hide the fact we were going through *that time of the month*.

At thirty-eight, I started dating my now-husband. We enjoyed each other and we did so many activities together such as frisbee golf, running, having dinner, local trips, just doing everything fun. We had an awesome time getting to know each other. I knew I was going to marry him three days into talking with him. He fit that saying, 'When you know you have met the one, you know.' That's exactly what happened. I asked him his thoughts on having kids and his ideas matched my own thoughts. If it happened, it happened but we were not going to put pressure on ourselves to have a child. When we decided to get married, I was forty.

When I was reaching my mid to upper thirties, my period was starting to change. I took that as the usual hormonal changes with age and the damage from the sporadic times I was on birth control. I would go a few months without my period then I would have periods sometimes twice a month. I would use a pad and a tampon to catch the heavy flow. At night I'd sleep on a towel or wake up in the middle of the night to change the overnight pad I was even doubling up. I even had a friend offer me her birthing underwear she was given after she had her baby because I was telling her I felt like my uterus was about to fall out of me when I had my period. Eventually, I noticed my periods were getting lighter and lighter. Again, I did not think anything about it. Then I became aware that my menstrual cycles disappeared altogether.

The last few times before my period completely disappeared, I felt like my uterus was going to explode. I had such a heavy flow that I had to wear two pads that I would change at a minimum, twice, in the middle of the night. I would wear the black pants and sit on a towel just in case there was leakage. After those four to five heavy months in a row, my period never came again. When I saw my doctor to ask what could be going on, the first test she ordered was a pregnancy test. I thought here it is, she is going to come back and say, 'CONGRATULATIONS you are pregnant!' but instead she said, seems like perimenopause has set in. My only perimenopause symptom was the absence of monthly periods. The first thought when she told me was "Well there goes the idea of having kids!" I took the news well. I was a little sad that I couldn't give my husband that kind of news and also sad that the chance of being a mum was clearly one hundred per cent gone.

My husband and I did try to have kids even after my perimenopause news. I took medication to stimulate egg production, bought ovulation sticks to make sure my eggs were ready and waiting, had sex in crazy positions to give the sperm a better path to swim to my egg. After a while, we went back to our thought that we were not going to stress ourselves over the pressure of having kids. We were not going to try other ways to have kids and we decided adopting was something we did not want to do as well. Kids were going to happen the natural way.

THE JUDGING EXPECTATIONS

As I reached a fifteen-year milestone in my career, I was still content in my profession. I noticed the demand from my career shifted. What began to change was what my supervisors perceived as my time availability. There were late afternoon meetings and weekend work. I would look at my co-workers who had families of two, three, five plus kids and I was the employee with zero kids. There was an assumption that I didn't have any obligations in the late night or over the weekends. Extra assignments were automatically assigned to me without asking if I was available. In the beginning, my supervisor I got the *courtesy ask* about my availability. They would ask each employee their availability for a late afternoon meeting or weekend sports coverage. I thought that was fair, so everyone had a chance to take opportunities or make some overtime. After a while though, I was the first one asked, while the employees with the kids were not asked at all. I felt I was being singled out because there is the assumption childless means no other obligations. I had no child to drive to sports or activities or recitals or whatever kids have. Did my supervisors think I sat around the house in my underwear with no life? I had a supervisor tell me he only worried about me if I worked sixty-one hours in a week. In reality, I had a busy life. When I was single, I had a busy life with my friends and having fun. Getting married and having a husband didn't change that life. I now have someone to share my full active life with. Childless does not mean lifeless and lifeless does not mean purposeless.

REPRESENTATION THROUGH STRENGTH

I did not miss out on anything in my life because I am not a mother. I actually think I lived life more because I was not a mother. I believe it is strong of me knowing that I chose to not pressure myself to have kids. My identity could have been intertwined and embedded within having a family and our roles to be the wife and a mother. By the time women hit their forties or once their kids are grown and old enough to take care of themselves, sometimes women lose their sense of purpose. I want to invite these women to take the opportunity to reinvent themselves, start a new chapter or finish one that was only a few words started.

NEVER SAY NEVER

When I was growing up, girls did not have the same chances to experience sports and build the strength and confidence they have now. It was more find a man, get married, have a kid, be a mother, and rely on your husband. Growing up, I experienced the pressure to disappear into the crowd and hide myself. I considered myself a shy kid, a quiet kid, but when physical activity was involved, I found my true self. When I engaged in sports, I experienced the happiest and most comfortable moments within myself. My protective father stopped me from being an athlete because I think the issue is often in my culture: the need to focus on my academics, get a respectable job, and anything that veered off that path was seen as a distraction, but I wanted so bad to be an athlete.

As I reached my forties, childless, I began to build the next chapter of my life. I was newly married, had a new job and a new house. A lot of new things and it was exciting. My life had a different feel, and I had a different focus and energy. I focused on living out a dream I had suppressed all my life. That dream was to be recognised as an athlete. My curiosity of being strong had grown bigger within me over the years. Strength carried a one-sided physical perception and as mentioned above, strength included being physically strong and mentally strong.

In March 2019, at forty-two, I tried something new, powerlifting. I did it for the sake of improving my health, but it added the curiosity of how strong I could become, building my own personal vision of an athlete. Thus, the passion for strength began. Just because I had hit perimenopause and was on my way to full menopause meant my refusal to disappear due to society's expectations became stronger as I did. Society's perception of what women can or cannot do as we reach our middle-age became more obvious to me. How we are done for because our bodies aren't as tight, our skin is not as supple and we have gone through things like marriages, divorces, surgeries, kids, no kids, multiple careers, makes us unmarketable.

Social media allows shows men leaving or divorcing the older woman to find a younger woman. Advertising even feeds into the fear of ageing by showing us items to erase our wrinkles, to use outside techniques to hide and prevent us from embracing and showing our age. We are so scared to age. The thought that when women hit a certain age that we are done for is a societal assumption I want to change. Ultimately, I feel like we allow ourselves to disappear from society when we don't own our strength. We allow ourselves to not be seen as much and become devalued because we have bought into the narrative that we do not have anything more to offer besides being a baby incubator, AND THAT THINKING IS SO WRONG!

As an Athletic Trainer I was considered a medical health professional, and I knew menopause has a different and vast array of effects on every woman. Menopause starts with a decrease in muscle mass, decrease in strength and bone density. With that knowledge in the back of my mind touching the thoughts of building my strength, it fuelled my power. Not only did I want to get strong to prevent breaking my hip if I lost my balance, but I also wanted to hold off the onset of other ailments that happen as I age.

Second to the health benefits of getting strong, I decided to build the representation I did not see of what an athlete was when I was a young girl. The challenge, how was I going to stretch my capabilities to become a strength athlete? First, I had to make the decision to look for a coach/personal trainer. I found one that helped me build my base of knowledge and technique so I could begin training as an athlete.

My first day at the specialised powerlifting and strongman gym, I met three women who were in their twenties and they were so strong. I watched one of them squat in the upper 200s and deadlift over 300 lbs. I was in awe. This was what I wanted to see. Strong women. What was missing was the representation of an older woman lifter. When we got to sit and talk, we clicked like we had known each other for years. One of the first questions they asked me was my age. I said forty-two. They were in shock. They could not believe I had an interest in powerlifting at my age. I educated them on why I wanted to lift. I told them I believe strength in women was important. I believed how strength gives women a confidence they never knew they had, that strength creates a different aura in a woman. We walk with our shoulders back; we have a 'Do not underestimate me' attitude. I loved these women, but they still weren't representative of me: a forty-two-year-old, childless woman who wanted to be strong as possible. I did not care about the judgments from others of my choosing strength as my way of fitness. All I wanted to do was train to get strong and compete, like an athlete would. In November 2019, I did a non-sanctioned powerlifting meet. After that, my mind shifted.

Besides learning powerlifting techniques, I learned more about my capabilities. My mind strength was getting built along with my muscles. The mould that I was put in as a young girl was breaking. I had a stronger mind and an able body. I found myself through the barbell. Lifting made me feel capable of doing something that I had wanted to do for almost a decade. The barbell keeps you wanting to get better and better, stronger and stronger. I knew I wanted MORE for my life.

Building my physical strength allowed me to believe I deserved more. As I said before, sports were something that I was not exposed to when I was younger. What I found in my forties was that my soul was waiting for me to unleash my inner strength. Having this strength allowed me to find my voice.

In my teens, I was holding myself back due to the expectations of my family. In my twenties, I was holding myself back due to the expectations from my family and society. In my thirties, I was holding myself back because I was getting too old to have the life I thought I wanted in my twenties. In my forties it was time to live in the now, learn from the past to move forward with the knowledge to know I am capable of whatever I choose for myself. Now my soul is awake and ready to go forward.

IRON TRUTH

I strength train and do strength sports not only for the mental benefits, but to put women's strength sports on the map. I know a lot of older women who see themselves as unseen and unheard, so I take up space and allow myself to be seen whilst guiding other women to do the same. I'm a different person since starting powerlifting and dabbling into strength sports. In the past, I would let supervisors speak condescendingly towards me because I did not feel strong enough to speak up for myself. I was also fearful to stand up for myself, refusing the extra hours and workload just because I was a childless woman who didn't have a family to get home to. In my past romantic relationships, I took on the persona of what they wanted me to be. I let society and other people's expectations dictate my life and what they thought I should be. When I started powerlifting, the level of confidence and courage began to rise. Now, I am bringing my confidence and voice together.

I am done making myself small for others for others to understand me and for me to fit in. I have had a power within me that has been stifled through decades, and generations of fear and cultural expectations. It was time to change the narrative of what I had been programmed to be and what was expected of me.

Sport has given me a unique perspective and a heightened awareness of my inner power. I learn more and more about myself taking part in a sport I enjoy and one which challenges me. Powerlifting allows me to face a wall that might have stopped me from trying something new and succeeding. I use strength as a platform to overcome self-doubt, low self-esteem, and low self-confidence. The lessons from powerlifting crossover from the platform to my life. I found more of myself through the barbell. Lifting made me feel capable of doing something that I had wanted to do for almost a decade. There is a saying I heard about powerlifting and strength sports 'The bar will tell you the truth.' I believe that. The iron not only tells you what you can, or you can't lift at the moment, it gives you the opportunity to reach for the possible. It takes work, but every step gets you stronger and stronger. It allowed me to do something that I never believed possible.

It would be very remiss of me to not talk about my Filipino background, and the unspoken expectations for Asian women was to stay fragile, stay quiet and remain unnoticed. I had great Filipino women to look up to in my family, but I wanted to add to that. I wanted more. What I looked for when it came to representation for me was a physically strong, confident, Asian woman. You can exercise but being 'too big' in the Asian culture is not feminine.

For years I lived a life that played toward the fear of disappointment. This fear held me back from embracing and accepting my strength. My strength is my courage. My strength is my POWER. Seeing a physical change in my body was just the tip of the iceberg. Society played on my fear and made me question my body and my capabilities. Getting stronger reminded me that I was worthy, and I possessed within me the confidence that kept me positive and moving forward.

If I were to choose between being silent and small versus big, taking up space and using my voice, I will always choose to get big. Powerlifting has helped me define my standard for myself. As women are trying to get smaller, I am trying to get as big as possible. Powerlifting demands I take up space and grow. Instead of competing with others, I compete with myself. My strength is measured by my capability and not my weight or my clothing size. The ability to gain strength through powerlifting encourages women to be bigger—and not just physically. The barbell does not care what size you are, what your nine to five job is, or if you have groomed yourself or not. It is between you and the bar. When your hands grasp the weight, it comes down to either you can lift the weight, or you cannot. Strength requires you to get stronger by confronting your familiar discomfort and accepting failures

Lessons from powerlifting extend way beyond the platform. Powerlifting helped me overcome the standards that were placed upon me and helped me be comfortable in my body. All my life, I was telling myself I needed to be smaller and thinner. I used to poke and prod and squeeze myself like a tomato to check ripeness. Now I feel myself to see how much my muscles have grown. I look in the mirror and give myself an approving head nod because I am loving my body. It looks so strong, and powerlifting gave me a stronger heart. When I feel strong and confident, it helps me support others achieve their goals. I get to share their excitement when they perform a successful lift. I get to hi-five women that I know that are stronger physically than me, but there is the camaraderie with my fellow competitors.

There is nothing to prove to others in powerlifting. All I know is that it took me over forty years to find what I needed in my life to overcome my past. Lifting weights helped me get through some depression and the complacency of life. I own who I am now. I own my power and strength, and it feels like me. Just me, and I have written my own standards and expectations. My choice. My Strength. I am purposely getting strong so I can help carry someone who feels they don't have the strength to be strong and who feels like they are unable to find themselves. I want to be there to help them get to their start line. Once I get them there, I will support them and encourage them, but it's up to them to take those steps forward.

When I am competing, I'm stretching my confidence and my capabilities. The mental shift towards myself brought with it a different kind of self-love and self-respect. The iron helped me outgrow and outperform the standards set upon me as a young child and young adult. I love myself more. I stopped comparing myself to others and I knew that there was more, and I could achieve it.

Fast forward two years, and I now hold a record in the State of Illinois for a deadlift of 402lbs as a Masters[1] athlete. I have competed in three powerlifting meets and two strongman competitions. Reaching forty-five years old, I decided I am going to change the idea that when you reach your forties, and are childless, along with reaching full-blown menopause, life is not over. Life has just taken a different path.

FULFILLED

When I got married at forty years old, I was still childless, by choice and by physiology. According to one of the doctors I saw, my egg production was of a sixty-year-old woman and the chance to get pregnant was slim. I was put on some medication to stimulate my egg production and the medication made me feel terrible. I knew my husband now wanted to be a father, and we agreed that we would give it a go for a year to try naturally and that we were not going to stress about it after that. I bought those ovulation sticks to check for those hormones and eggs to drop and be ready. After sex, I would situate my body against the headboard, so my legs were up in the air. I would lay there scrolling on my phone for thirty minutes to help the sperm swim up to my eggs. There were even times, I would do it for forty-five minutes. My husband and I continued to live our lives and without stressing about it. Our decision to let nature take its course did not deprive me of sex. I did my part to fulfil my reproductive purpose without any pressure. We wanted to enjoy each other in our young marriage and that was what mattered to us. Yes, we live our lives without the demand of parenthood. We work, travel, go out to dinner when we want, and we talk about how we do not stress going from weekend sports or activities. We have absolutely no regrets.

---

1   The IWF (International Weightlifting Federation) categorises a master's athlete thirty-five years of age and up. https://www.teamusa.org/usa-weightlifting/weightlifting101/age-groups

I get asked if we are still going to try. People have said that we should keep trying and we would be amazing parents. My response to that "Meh, what happens, happens." My husband and I are happy with what we have, and we do not live an unfulfilled life. If a child happens to come, awesome. We will love it and be the best parents we can be.

REFLECTION
Strength is Universal.

What many cultures fail to realise is that there are a lot of versions of people and life plans. When it comes to women, we are multi-faceted, multi-layered, and are different shapes and sizes and people judge us. We are too big for people's liking, too small for people's liking, too this and too that. It can be exhausting to fall into the "shoulda," "woulda", "coulda" thinking. If I had kids, people would judge how I was parenting. I don't have kids, and I get judged. If I have a partner, I will get judged. What I do with my life, is my life. The strength that I have now allows me to overlook the judging eyes. Culture will continue to pressure me to do things that they want me to do.

I was asked once during a podcast interview, when I was going to stop doing the powerlifting or training to lift big weights. Also, if I was afraid about becoming too manly. Why is the first thing people think about when women lifting, is that we will look manly? Do people ever think that a woman lifting just wants to be strong and having some muscle is just a result of that strength? People do not realise the reason for strength is universal. Strength in the physical sense is not the only trait someone can have.

Since menopause has set in, I accepted that my chances of motherhood have become zero to none. I am considered a middle-aged or older woman now, but that does not mean I should not continue to pursue my hidden potentials. I am multi-layered, and I choose to explore those hidden potentials. As menopause settles in a variety of ways for women at various times, I now have a strong community to interact with, and to keep my mental state churning. First, I want to have a strong quality of life as I age. If I fall, I want to be able to get myself up physically. I do not want to lose the power to challenge my mind and lifting has helped me with that. Do you know how hard bar math is? Second, I want to take every opportunity to put older women athletes in the spotlight.

Women experiencing menopause does not automatically mean the end of life. We are women, strength athletes or not, and we are amazing women. It is often forgotten that older women are serious athletes. Just because our bodies have gone through changes, does not mean we cannot become accomplished athletes. Many athletes have overcome difficulties in life. Overcoming is a part of what makes us strong. Physical strength in the older female population is not going away. We are not a demographic to be overlooked. There are women in their sixties holding world records in strength sports. We are here to celebrate our strengths. The younger demographic may get all the glory, but the older women are coming to join the party.

I want to increase the number of opportunities for older women to embrace their physical strength and not to be afraid of it. This mindset shows that anybody can be strong no matter what is happening with their body physiologically. Anybody can have a chance to build what they want.

When I heard about being a contributor to this book, I had to think long and hard about contributing. I never thought about menopause being a big part of my life because it is just a part of my life. I thought about the life experiences that come along with menopause. Once I may have thought that I was a bad person and there must be a reason I am not being blessed with children. With no regret or guilt, I do not focus on societies pressures of what a women's life should look like. I have developed a passion to encourage and inspire women to realise their identity is not wholly tied to being a mother. I know women whose one goal is to have kids and will do what they need to do to add a child to their lives. IVF, surrogates, adopting, etc. I remember having a conversation years before I got married that I should think about adoption because there are lots of kids that need a good parent. They thought I would be a great parent because I was fun. Parenting needs a lot more than me being fun.

I am worth a story of my own. I want other women to believe, they are worthy of their own story as well. Our stories build role models for young girls that don't see an array of role models. To show there are other options in life and if someone does not want kids that's ok. My hope is to inspire more diverse participation in strength sports. I want women to see that strength is not saved for the young. Strength is universal.

Reflections

Reflections

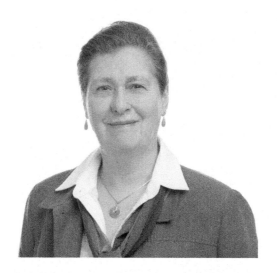

ANN MOIR-BUSSY
AUSTRALIA

Dr Ann Moir-Bussy is an educator, counsellor, transformative life coach, consultant and best-selling author.

She initially trained as a teacher and worked in schools throughout Australia including many Indigenous schools in the Northern Territory. She also trained students in counselling practice in Australia and Hong Kong.

Ann established her own business Embrace Life Now and also has an exclusive program for women moving through midlife into the afternoon of life. She has a series of podcasts called Alchemy in the Midlife Kitchen.

Ann has developed effective and powerful ways to facilitate change and healing, enabling clients to be the best possible version of themselves, able to attain their goals and dreams. She believes in a holistic approach that embraces all aspects of life and integration of mind, body, and spirit. In addition to this, Ann is a Reiki Master and practices Qigong and meditation daily.

Websites

www.embracelifenow.com.au

https://annmoirbussy.com

"Wake at dawn with a winged heart and give thanks for another day of loving."
– Kahil Gibran

Chapter Eight

THE JOURNEY OF TRANSFORMATION AND INITIATION: ALCHEMY IN THE MID-LIFE KITCHEN

INTRODUCTION

My life journey has taken so many routes, detours, wrong turnings, mountains and valleys. I remember when I was teaching in Hong Kong, I had the opportunity to go to Beijing and climb part of the Great Wall of China. The higher we climbed the more spectacular the views and our perspective encompassed vistas we had never imagined possible. A similar experience was in Australia and we reached the top of Mt Kosciusko, where again, we were absorbed into a timeless and all-embracing universe that takes the breath away. Moments of delight and transformation that enabled us to view this life journey from above, as it were, and though difficult to put into words, makes it possible to view the transitions, endings and beginnings of life in a new light.

And so, my passage into and through menopause only takes meaning against the interconnection of people, and events who were all part of the journey, intertwined with other transitions that life afforded us, and viewed from multiple perspectives.

THE BEGINNING

Just over eighty years ago, early in World War II, my father had been called up to serve. He took a weekend to see my mother and I was conceived. Little did she know then that it would be almost four years before she saw him again and that he would be a prisoner of war in Changi, in Singapore, under the Japanese. I was born on the 2nd March 1942, in Bournemouth, England. My father had met Australian soldiers in the prison camp and on his return, they talked of emigrating, and in February 1949, we left for a new home in Australia – the first big transition, and adventure.

At age eleven, I found myself in puberty, and the monthly pattern of pain and heavy bleeding began, and while I had become responsible for younger siblings, I was also drawn into a different lifestyle. My parents had a strong faith and post war we "adopted" a Japanese child and began writing and sending gifts and clothes. It was a strong missionary era and we became imbued with this philosophy, so much so that I wanted to be a missionary and at twelve years of age joined a secondary school which trained and prepared young girls for this life. I was enthusiastic and entered wholeheartedly into the regime of hard physical work, study and prayer. Little by little as I conformed to what was required, I began to lose my spontaneity, and strove to "fit in," but this did not diminish the desire to serve.

At the conclusion of secondary schooling, I was formally accepted into the missionary group and in further training, learned more about the 'spirituality of the heart.' At the same time, my parents decided to commit some years of their life to also working as lay missionaries in Papua New Guinea. I was trained as a teacher and in my early twenties became a 'mother' and teacher in a boarding school in Alice Springs – in Central Australia. In those days it was a very remote place and the twenty-four girls I became responsible for, aged from five years to fourteen years all came from far away cattle stations. I slept in a small room off the dormitory and became "mum" and "dad" in all ways, alongside being a teacher by day, and living in the community. It was during those early years I had a sense that while this was all decent work and I'd conformed to the outer demanding work, there must be something more. The monthly cycle became more painful, but it was something we learned to endure!

(An aside, some of those Indigenous girls, now married themselves and in mid-life and beyond, still keep in touch and we had a great reunion may years later when I went back to work as a counsellor and consultant in the Northern Territory).

Postings to different schools, including Indigenous schools in remote parts of the Northern Territory, were all aspects of this 'missionary' work. As I neared my forties, an inner unfolding began to take place and an exhaustion began to set in. It seemed I was entering a dark tunnel and there was no way out, no light to guide me. At that time, I knew little about psychology, until I was introduced to Carl Jung and his appreciation of the symbolic life. Perimenopause was close (though I didn't realise it then), as periods became heavier and I was bleeding often and also haemorrhaging. Finally, I had to be taken to the city and told I would need a hysterectomy. Looking back, I realise the psychological implications of this, as my feminine spirit had been crushed and I had been moulded into a masculine system of power. But more of that soon as it is so important to acknowledge we ourselves are complicit in this process, and the stories that follow will demonstrate this.

AT THE THRESHOLD OF MID-LIFE

All the physical symptoms awakened me to the fact that I was nearing fifty and a new phase was about to begin. I could no longer continue with the same driven way of being, and while the hysterectomy meant that menopause was not quite the same, there were still obvious reactions. The very term menopause became for many women a very negative term. Bonnie Horrigan has authored a book Red Moon Passage (1996) – a term she coined for menopause, a word she notes is coined from the Greek word *meis* meaning "moon" and the French word *pause* meaning "pause". In other words, it is the cessation of menstruation, and hence, the cessation of the ability to give birth to new life.

There is no further meaning attached – it's the end or the stopping and infers that there is nothing beyond that. And so many women took it at that and ceased to live a joyful and fruitful life. Fortunately, we know differently now, and that one ending heralds a new beginning. The morning of life now awakens us to the afternoon of life, and menopause signals that we are standing on the threshold. Horrigan interviewed eight extraordinary women, and I have found much inspiration from their questioning of the status quo and the deep inner listening to their own intuition and their choice to step through the gate into their own mid-life journey.

As I stood on the threshold I too, found myself questioning the status quo and wondering how to find the way to consciously enter this new phase – a journey or transition that took me eight years.

ENTERING THE ALCHEMICAL KITCHEN

I stood on the threshold and I was terrified. I had a lot of experience but it was all tied up with the roles I had taken on and what I thought had been expected of me. My intuitive inner wisdom had long been silenced and buried, so much so that I did not trust my own voice. As I hesitated on the threshold, two guides came – a Jungian Analyst and a Spiritual Guide, and gently nudged me to the entrance.

You might be wondering why I called it the Alchemical Kitchen. Alchemy, as you may know, is a very ancient science with its origins stemming from the ancient civilisations of Egypt, China and Babylonia, where the knowledge was passed on to the Greeks and the Romans. The Greek philosophers had a strong influence on the foundation of Western Alchemy. And true alchemy involved both practice and study in a true 'holistic' sense. While the very ancient traditions were concerned with transmutation and the focus on searching for a method of the transmutation of base metals into gold, it quickly became much more concerned and involved with the deep philosophy of the transmutation of the soul.

In 200 BC the Egyptians spoke of *al = the* and *chemia = the black land* or the science of black earth or prima matter. Those motivated by only material gold found the writings confusing. Much visual imagery and symbolism was used and this is what found its way into the work on psychological transformation, especially in the work of Carl Jung who, in 1944 published his study on *Psychology and Alchemy*. He discovered in the images in dreams of his patients that symbolic images from alchemy also appeared, even though the patients know nothing of the alchemical work.

As I worked with the dark night within me and began to unravel the layers especially through the images in my dreams, the inner work was indeed similar to that of the alchemist, a sacred work of transformation and a deep search for the ultimate value in life. Like the alchemist, it was a solitary work. The alchemist worked mainly alone in a laboratory that was also an oratory – a place of prayer and solitude.

There are many beautiful images in the literature of alchemists working in the laboratory, (See Alchemy – *The Medieval Alchemists and their Royal Art* by Johannes Fabricius, 1976) gathering and separating the raw material, preparing it for being sealed in the retort and providing just the right amount of air, the right amount of heat and endless patience as he separated the dross from the ore. Here is not the place to explore in depth any more of alchemy - except to say it becomes a powerful symbol for what needs to happen as we approach mid-life and go through the transformation of leaving behind youth and the morning of life and entering the afternoon of life whilst embracing the process of gaining new wisdom.

The alchemist's approach to knowledge was holistic, seeking inner gold rather than the secularised approach of so many modern tertiary institutions which advocate outer achievement and outer appearances. It was a process of inner transformation.

How do we know we are ready for this? Fortunately, for us as women our body wakes us up to this time of change with the gradual ceasing of menstruation or being thrust into it with a hysterectomy, and the often many uncomfortable side effects of out of sync hormones, mood swings, tiredness, irritability, weight gain, restlessness and so on. For me it was also accompanied by a deep questioning of what had been the status quo, and the surgery followed by chronic fatigue. For many other women it might be children leaving home, divorce, arguments and work. I had begun this journey while still within the missionary group, and while I knew from my dreams and inner work that something had to change, the fear of 'what' and 'where' was strong. I read, studied, prayed, and tried to understand more but something was missing. There seemed to be some unnamed inner potential that was imprisoned within, something that in all the outer tears, was crying to be released. I loved the missionary work but struggled to find another way.

Have you too, lived a full morning of life, juggling family and career, relationships, success or not? You have gained lots of wisdom, knowledge, experience – all of which is wonderful. Maybe, you have also made mistakes or taken wrong turnings or fateful detours. But now, in midlife, your body is telling you that "something has to change" and - you are standing on the threshold of the most important journey of your life and the discovery of a "Great Work" – your transformation of all your morning of life experiences into gold for the afternoon of your life. How sad that across much of our Western culture menopause is treated as a purely physical and emotional experience, and the loss of youth and the ability to give birth, but that is only one dimension and very few have the words to think of it also as a spiritual passage, and the entrance to a whole new level of reality.

CHALLENGES – THE BELIEFS AND PATTERNS THAT WOUNDED OUR SOUL

In the era in which I had been growing through the morning of life, the world had become dominated by masculine principles which valued competition, achievement, success, being on top of things, keeping up with the status quo – the 'shoulds' and 'oughts' and conforming to expectations. Even though there was an attempt to set one's own expectations, little did most of us realise that these expectations were set largely by this masculine dominated society. And from the time I was twelve I had also lived in the shadow of a church that was very patriarchal in its approach.

This is not a condemnation of men – it is about the fact that so many men and women did not know how to balance both masculine and feminine principles within each of us. If the masculine is one-sided, it becomes harsh and dominating, and if the feminine is one-sided, it lacks the ability to stand up for oneself or to speak with one's own voice.

So, as I struggled with the physical changes, and the need to have a hysterectomy, I felt as though my whole feminine being was about to be raped, dismembered. As I studied more of Jungian psychology, I also became aware of the great archetypal myths that brought some understanding to this part of the journey. And what I learned, more than anything else, was that menopause asks us to **LISTEN – to listen to our body and our soul.**

I learned from Dante, the pilgrim poet of the 12th century, who found his way back to the Light and to his Soul and beloved only after a journey out the dark wood where he awoke to find himself totally lost. He was in midlife, and as he tried to force his way out, he was pushed back and his way out was blocked by a leopard, a lion and a she-wolf. As he said, *"How I got there I do not know, I must have become sleepy and strayed from the path of truth."* As he called out for help, he was sent a guide, the poet Virgil, who said

"But you must journey down another road, if ever you hope to leave this wilderness."

And he learned that he must go into the depths of the underworld (hell), then climb the mountain of Purgatory, before he could find his way to his own home within himself. And the message he was given:

"Because your question searches for deep meaning, I shall explain in simple words, A man must stand in fear of just those things that truly have the power to do us harm, of nothing else, for nothing else is fearsome."

As I wrestled and struggled with dark thoughts, and fear and those things that had the power to harm me, my guides patiently walked with me and let me rage and sob and helped with the imagery in my dreams that led me to see, I needed to find a way to embrace the feminine and the masculine. I needed to let go of the story that I had been living which was not my story but the story of the collective masculine, and to rewrite my own narrative.

Eight years may seem a long time, but like the alchemist, patience was needed, to allow what had been buried in the unconscious of my psyche, to emerge, to be cleansed, to be transformed.

Another beautiful image came from the Descent of the Goddess, the story of Inanna, goddess of the sky, who went to the underworld as her sister's husband had died and lost everything. They took her clothes, her body, her life, and only then with help of her aides is she reborn. Menopause can be the call to go deeper within ourselves and to find the wise woman within, which can only happen when we see what needs to be sacrificed and left behind so that we can move forward.

We can't always leave the story we have been living in one leap. Even today, menopause has been silenced in so many ways, and if not silenced, dominant voices have focussed on the physical, not only the collective voices of others, but also of social media, voices which urge a woman to return to her youth, to try and find ways to deny the body changing and hide the beauty of what is emerging within her. Many of the patterns that have wounded our souls are so deep, just like a lawn that has been trodden over in a path through the middle till there are only grooves of dirt and the grass is no longer there. If we want it to be renewed, we have to find and walk a different path.

BEING A HANDLESS MAIDEN

The above stories are about transformation and they all made sense to me. What I discovered, was that I needed to understand the physiological, psychological and spiritual aspects of menopause, which I was thrust into with the hysterectomy. Some women may experience only the physical, some may actually not experience any of the changes and others may experience all three. Maybe a lot of what a woman will experience will have much to do with their constitution in the morning of life, both emotionally and spiritually and may also be to do with the path to which one has been called. My early training had prepared me to some degree and enabled me to be open to the dark night. It didn't, however, make it any easier. There was loss of the reproductive function, scars to the physical body and loss and change to physical beauty, and then the crossing into the afternoon of life. And when I chose to leave the security and conformity of the missionary life, there lay before me a great unknown.

I was not leaving behind the 'spirituality of the heart' - and as Dante was told the message was "You must journey down another road." I had to find a new way to live and to allow the deep feminine intuition to give birth to the wise woman within.

In her book *Women Who run with the Wolves*, Clarissa Pinkola Estés (1992) uses myths and stories with vivid imagery to help us understand the journey of our psyche and consciousness throughout the stages of our life. She has gathered stories from many traditions and uses the healing medicine of stories to awaken us to our need to connect with the wise and wild woman within.

Some of the above stories I've talked about represent that journey into the underworld, or inward journey or looking into oneself and taking stock. I found that one of the best stories that most represents our journey into and through menopause is the story of *The Handless Maiden*.

It's one of those stories where you find you actually become a participant in her test of endurance. It's the story about a woman's initiation into the underground forest, where she learns 'endurance' – a word which means we become strong, sturdy, and strengthened – we are not just surviving, we are actually in the process of creating something new and beautiful. And we learn this in nature – like the underground forest. In this story, her descents (there are more than one) into the forest resemble the imagery of alchemical change. Or our encounter with earth, air, water and fire.

As with many other stories, the maiden lives alone with her father and mother, and there was always challenging work to make ends meet. The important thing to remember in these myths about a woman's development is that all the characters represent aspect of a woman's psyche. The male characters represent in some form a woman's *animus* and often in the early stages of a woman's life this masculine principle within a woman is not developed or is neglected. But more of that later.

The family is poor and the devil in guise of an old man, promises him wealth if he can have the first thing he sees behind the mill. The farmer thinks of his apple tree but to his horror it is his daughter sweeping the yard. The devil demands the girl.

When the devil came to collect her, she bathed, dressed in a white robe and stood within a circle of white chalk. He was thrown back by a powerful force and could not reach her. She is left for a while and dared not wash again until her hair became matted and her skin and clothes all dirty. When he came again, she wept so much that her tears ran down her arms and hands and they became clean and again he could not touch her. So, his order was "Chop off her hands so I can come near her." And he continued, "If you don't, everything here will die including you and all the fields."

The young girl had been taught that submission and obedience to her father were most important, and though she was not happy she agreed. It reminded me of the times I to submitted to patriarchal decisions, believing they knew best.

As we begin our journey through puberty into adulthood, which part of us makes a 'bargain,' or surrenders part of our deep intuitive, creative and instinctive life in order to please someone else – and usually we don't realise it. How many women have come to me and told how they have devoted so many years to their family, their children, their husband, or their work, and now they feel confused and lost, or handless? They don't know how to give love to themselves or have compassion and care for themselves.

The father, symbolising the part of our psyche that is supposed to guide us in the outer world, does not know the world of the soul, or how to guide his daughter, so she is endangered. But no girl can remain innocent forever and part of her growing to maturity is through suffering and betrayal and vulnerability and our maiden in the story, leaves home and wanders through the forest.

I certainly wandered in the forest.

The girl's transformation and initiation begin when she comes across a beautiful garden filled with pear trees. It belongs to a king and there is a moat around the castle. Some inner desire and need took hold of her, the moat is drained, and she walks across. A pear tree bends to her and she is finally able to eat a little fruit. A gardener had seen it and tells the king who the next night watches himself and becomes the one who supports her for the next phase of her journey, which also includes another descent into the forest.

There are so many images in this story, but space does not allow us to go into full detail. For me, the image of being handless, of allowing our deep knowing to be cut off, in service of what we think is a greater good is a powerful one, and when we begin to recognise this, there are tears for we must grieve. We have the choice then to give up or to remember we have feet and to move forward, even though it is still a time of wandering.

This journey of menopause is where we are transformed from the handless maiden to the woman who finds her own voice and brings love and compassion to herself; her transforming and her initiation into her ageing and full womanhood. Our hands grow back and our ability to nurture all aspects of life blossoms.

FOREVER PREGNANT, FOREVER GIVING BIRTH, FOREVER, A VIRGIN

As I continued this inner and lonely outer journey, I came across another wonderful book by Marion Woodman titled *The Pregnant Virgin*. It is a book for women in mid-life and is about the struggle for a woman to become conscious – it is about the wisdom of the body, initiation, ritual and dreams and it is about our relationship and search for personal identity. It is also the celebration of the feminine in men and women. She uses the beautiful imagery of the metamorphosis of the caterpillar to the chrysalis to butterfly as being akin to a woman in midlife when we find ourselves again in the chrysalis and life as we have known it is over and we are basically alone. We can no longer be who we were, and we don't yet know who we will become.

A woman moving through menopause said to me recently in a session, "I'm confused, I don't know who I am anymore, I feel lost and I'm scared. I find myself wanting to run away, and I do it by getting into relationships where I'm pleasing men again..."

This is the chrysalis and if a woman is prepared to be with that fear of the unknown and let the transformation take place, she will get closer to her inner virgin – "she who is one-in-herself," forever open to new life, new possibilities, to her own truth.

Mary Esther Harding (1888-1971) was an English Jungian analyst who explored the psychology of women and believed that a woman needed to achieve virginity by being one-in-herself. She wrote:

"She is virgin, even while being goddess of love. She is essentially one-in-herself. She bears her divinity in her own right... The woman who is virgin, does what she does – not of a desire to please, not to be liked, not to be approved, even by herself; but because what she does is true" (M.E. Harding, 1990, p. 125)

Being one-in-herself, the woman is free to be pregnant with creativity, with the new life in her that is becoming, and give birth to the beauty and love and deep intuition within her. Welcome to the most beautiful part of your life. Having been through the physical, emotional, psychological and spiritual descent/s in the forest or the underworld, you can now bring forth wisdom, leadership and the ability to bring about change and influence.

Another feminist philosopher and psychoanalyst, Lucie Irigaray, claimed that virginity is a metaphor of integrity and spirituality, alluding "to the capacity of gathering, keeping and transforming energy of one's own" (Irigaray, 2008a, p.105)

Alchemy in the Mid Life Kitchen is the journey and process of being forever pregnant, forever giving birth and forever a virgin. It is also where you bring all those early experiences and transform them into gold – it is a journey into your inner world alongside the journey through what is happening in your body through menopause.

THE BLACK NUBIAN WOMAN – LEARNING COMPASSION FOR YOUR WOUNDED SELF IN MENOPAUSE

As I said earlier, a great beauty about menopause is that it is a passage into more depth and internal riches in oneself, especially if we enter the transformative power of the Alchemical Kitchen. And stories are indeed powerful – especially if we can notice where we become part of the story. Learning deep self-compassion during menopause was not easy for me, as I had been trained for so long to endure things, and not in a positive way, but by ignoring the pain or 'putting up with it."

A story that Laurens Van der Post collected in Africa has great teaching in it and transmitted values and wisdom that taught me a lot about this self-compassion. It was the story of the *Black Nubian Woman*. It is another story of feminine initiation where we learn to trust our own guidance and nature. As with many stories it happened a long, long time ago or maybe yesterday or last week. And it is about a beautiful black Nubian woman who walked through her village in a beautiful red toga and carrying a basket on her head. She had a magnificent necklace of ju-ju beads as it was the custom for all the women to wear such necklaces. Women still wear such necklaces today.

All the other women were jealous of her because of the beauty of her necklace and the grace and dignity with which she walked and they promised each other that one day they would take this necklace from her. She could hear them whispering as she walked through the village and they avoided her and were not friendly and her heart ached as she wondered what she had done to make them exclude her.

Each week they went down to the river to wash their clothes and they would laugh and splash as they waited for them to dry on the river bank. This time they said to her, "Oh we have been unkind to you, why don't you come and play with us?" She was touched and then noticed they didn't have on their necklaces and asked then what they had done so she could put hers there too.

"Oh, we made an offering to the river gods and we threw our necklaces to them with a prayer."

She thought this was a kind thing to do and so took off her necklace, prayed to the river gods and threw it in where it went down, down, deep into the mud.

The women laughed and made fun of her and said "Do you think we would be so stupid and pulled their necklaces out from the mud, washed them and put them on and left her.

Left alone she wept and prayed to the gods and goddesses to bring it back for her, and as she was crying, she heard a voice say, "Dive in, dive in." Hesitant at first, till she heard it again and with courage she dived down to the depths of the river bed and as the mud cleared, she saw a very old woman sitting there with oozing sores all over her. And she heard the woman say, "Lick my sores, lick my sores." The black Nubian woman felt sorry for the old woman and went down on her knees and began to lick one of the sores, and immediately her face became clear and beautiful.

Does it remind you of the princess who had to kiss the frog in order to get her ball back?

Suddenly there was a terrible noise and the demon of the river was shouting. "I can smell a young woman, where is she?" The old woman quickly hid her under her clothes and told the demon that she had gone another way and off he went looking for her. When it became quiet again, she pulled the woman out and then dug down and brought up an exquisite necklace made of silver and gold, crystals and diamond, and then put it round her neck.

She clapped her hands and the woman was back on the river bank and then a beautiful white basket and a beautiful white toga. She dressed in them and as she looked into the now clear river, she saw a reflection of herself and she saw the soul of herself.

What a wonderful image for loving, cleansing and bringing self-compassion to all parts of ourself, and especially those wounded parts which graphically can seem like "oozing sores." Again, we do this in the alchemical kitchen as we lovingly leave behind what is no longer needed and embrace all aspects of the woman within and allow both the wise woman and the wild woman to emerge, the woman who embraces her instinctual self, claims her passion and her vibrancy and takes the transformed silver and gold into her new way of being.

RECLAIM MENOPAUSE, CLAIM YOUR CROWN AND BECOME THE CRONE

Menopause gives the place and space for a woman to give birth to the wild woman and the wise woman. You can't have one without the other because they are ONE, they are twins. We are born with the seeds of wholeness within us. So, what happened and why do so many women deny the gift of who they really are?

Unfortunately, some women see this giftedness as a curse, not a blessing because from childhood we are often trained to FIT IN, to be normal. But being normal or normalcy is an enemy of giftedness and it encourages us to deny the gift of who we are as a woman.

Recently I came across Estés book *The Dangerous Old Woman* (2010) an Audio CD on Sounds True and she tells the stories and myths herself with such feeling and knowingness. She notes that if we reclaim the purpose of our menopause, accept and embrace the transition and the transformation, then we can break free from normalcy, listen to, and allow the wise and wild woman. – "the dangerous old woman" as she calls her, to find expression within us.

I love this image and it is such a powerful one for women to recognise – *the dangerous old woman.* Throughout history the masculine system of power became more dominant and denigrated women and denied the sacred experience of menopause. They didn't want to know about it as they we afraid of the own inability to relate and to connect to their own anima – their inner feminine.

Long, long ago the word dangerous had a very different meaning to what we mean by its use today

Dangerous meant *to protect* – and Estés says that we were never meant to harm certain things – so 'don't stand in my danger as I will do everything to protect her'. The dangerous old woman is not a person who insults, harms or belittles others.

Literally it meant that you are standing in my danger, you are encroaching on my aura surrounding me, and I will protect that fiercely, I will defend it, do anything to protect it if you get in the way of the truth and beauty of all living creatures.

The dangerous old woman is the one who looks after those who have been conquered and raises them up again.

She is observant, and experienced, and she will protect anything that has goodness in it anything she breathes on and she will bring it back it to life. I am reminded of one of Estés first stories in *Women who run with the Wolves*, where she tells the story of La Loba (1992,2008, p. 23), who gathers the bones of wolves, sings over them and brings them back to life. She collects and preserves that which is in danger of being lost to the world. She preserves and cares for feminine intuition and feminine tradition. She is in our deepest soul psyche – the wise and wild woman within us who was often imprisoned within us in the first half of our life.

We have seen the masculine system rape our earth, tear down trees, dry up rivers, fight wars and seek power in so many ways. We now have to become 'dangerous' ourselves in the true meaning of the word – protectors of life in all its forms. We learn to be 'dangerous' but dependable. Our home is in the soul.

The dangerous old woman is the twin of the wise old woman and wisdom is many things.

What is WISDOM? It's not to do with years or how old we are. Some old women do not have wisdom and some small children have a deep wisdom. Wisdom is about knowing the world, knowing the creative force, knowing the soul and knowing pragmatic things. Wisdom is in tune with the soul and grows with times of silence, meditation, and solitude, which is why the time of menopause is so important.

Wisdom is *what works* for the soul, the spirit, the heart, the mind the body *in this moment* and for *all moments*. Wisdom is that which you love and that which loves the world.

And so, wisdom can be unpredictable because creation is not static. We don't suddenly find wisdom and that's it. As I said with the 'dangerous old woman' there is not normalcy and so with wisdom, there is constant evolution and becoming.

Menopause is where we claim our CROWN and begin the journey of ageing and becoming the CRONE – the woman who crowns her wisdom. We befriend the *HAG* and call on Hygiea – the goddess of wisdom. And we remain the maiden, the Virgin, the woman who is one-in-herself. We call back the dismembered parts of ourselves – we are old and we are young at the same time. We are pregnant and we are giving birth.

PUTTING MENOPAUSE BACK ON THE MAP

Now is the time for women to initiate women and we can only do this if we have been through our own transformation and initiation. Women going into menopause can initiate girls going into puberty for in one the cycle has gone full circle and in the other the blood is beginning to flow. If menopause is something to be feared, it could be that we have not been mentored well. In menopause we grieve the young girl, but wisdom knows she is still incorporated within us.

We go alone into menopause because it is a deep spiritual initiation and as in the alchemical kitchen, we are the ones who watch and care for this transition and see all those experiences that led up to this moment transform into gold for the rest of our life. Alchemists had a support worker and we can be that for each other too. But we have to do the inner work. If enough women do this, we can change the world. We must not be afraid to speak about it, to challenge the stereotypical social media jargon and the way the pharmaceutical companies speak about menopause as though a woman will be fixed if she 'pops a pill.' And we must not ignore the cycles of life.

Menopause is not a disease – it is a transition, a gateway into a beautiful unfolding, creativity, zest, and where we leave behind what is no longer needed and embrace our deep instinctual, emotional, spiritual and physical self.

I want to finish with telling you about Alice Walker and her wonderful book of poetry, *Hard Times Require Furious Dancing (2010)*. In it she has one poem that speaks to all of us as we pass through menopause into the afternoon of life and it is titled *Calling all Grand Mothers* (2010, pp.30-32).

She challenges women to step up and out and to take their place as leaders and as wise women in the world. As I have said earlier, we have to remember who we are and who we are becoming and we must take on that role of mentoring those women who are coming after us. We must stop hiding with false humility, or with an excuse that we have nothing to say. Share what you have learned and radiate that vibrant energy of the Crone in whatever way you can. No one else can share your experience and wisdom for you are one-of-a-kind.

So, let us stop being normal – let us be who we were born to be!

REFERENCES

Estés, Clarissa Pinkola (1992, 2008) *Women who run with the wolves*, Rider, UK.

Estés, Clarissa Pinkola (2010) *Dangerous Old Woman: Myths and Stories about the Wise Woman Archetype.* Audio CD. Sounds True

Fabricius, J. (1976) *Alchemy – The Medieval Alchemists and their Royal Art.* The Aquarian Press, Copenhagen.

Harding, M.E. (1990) *Women's Mysteries, Ancient and Modern.* Boston, Shambhala, p. 125).

Horrigan, B.J. (1996) *Red Moon Passage – the power and wisdom of menopause.* Thorsons, London.

Irigaray, L. (2008) *Conversations.* London. Continuum. P, 105.

Walker, A. (2010) *Hard times require furious dancing.* New World Library, Novato, California

Von Franz, M-L. (1980) Alchemy – *An introduction to the symbolism and the psychology.* Inner City Books: Toronto, Canada

Walker, A. (2010) Calling all Grand Mothers, in Walker, A. *Hard Times Require Furious Dancing,* New World Library, Novato, CA. pp. 30-32

Woodman, Marion (1985) The Pregnant Virgin – A Process of Psychological transformation. Inner City Books, Toronto.

Reflections

Reflections

Reflections

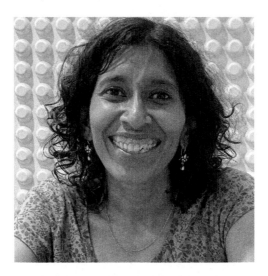

MAGGIE INBAMUTHIAH
INDIA

Maggie Inbamuthiah is an entrepreneur, community builder, a vocal enthusiast for diversity and social equity, and a lifelong traveller. She curates the DEI and Global Well-being networks at Executive Networks working with HR leaders across Fortune 500 companies, while also offering consulting services in the field of ESG via Handful of Sky.

During the weekends you will find her hiking taking people on her soul-venture Happifeet. Maggie is the co-founder of Mandram, a non-profit working to bring Indic languages back into mainstream dialogue.

She is also a Yoga teacher in the Krishnamcharya tradition with a deep interest in holistic living. She writes regularly in her blog site on various topics from travel to mountaineering to philosophy.

Maggie was previously the head of AnitaB.org India and collaborated with women in tech in India to run the Asia's largest technology conference for women, the Grace Hopper Celebration India.

Maggie lives in India, close to the Himalayas.

Chapter Nine

THE PATH TO MENOPAUSE

A wonder woman is writing this chapter; a woman wondering what her menopause will be like.

I have started hearing anecdotes from my friends. Some are concerning; some sound as easy as a cake walk. But I don't yet have a firsthand experience of menopause. The anxiety and fear about what's in store make me nervous every time I sweat (pun intended), and that I think needs a chapter in itself. Given this, I wonder, what am I doing in this book. If you too are wondering my dear reader, let me offer this. According to the UN[1], there are 3.95 billion women in this world, representing 49.58 per cent of the entire population. Out of this, 984 million women are aged fifty and above, most of whom we can assume are going through or have gone through menopause. The population of women in the age of fifteen – forty-nine is then in the menstrual age. This number is 1.9 billion or 49.18 per cent of the entire population of women. Mine is a voice from this pool narrating the journey towards menopause; a journey filled with anxiety, aversion and complete lack of knowledge and hence preparedness.

---

1   UN – United Nations

The first time I heard the word menopause with reference to me was at forty. It was a jolt. I was trekking the Himalayas; my first ever; with a group of strangers, first ever as well. After a day of climbing, we were sitting in the dining tent and chatting. I lightheartedly threw this question to the group, "What do you think happens to women in their forties?"

The eighteen-year-old medical student in the group was quick to respond, "Menopause."

I was speechless. Never mind that I had a well thought out follow through, that involved women having the time and space to find themselves and pursue their passion in their forties, as the kids turned older. The world just viewed women as models when young, then as mothers and then menopausal, it seemed.

What I remember vividly from that exchange is my aversion towards the word menopause. I didn't want it. Not so soon.

There were three things that stood between me and the dreaded M-word.

1. Menopause meant old.
2. Menopause meant useless and unattractive.
3. Menopause meant a difficult transition and I had no idea what it was like.

Growing old and menopause are two inevitable things women seemed to run away from and I was no exception.

As I ran in the opposite direction of ageing, I hit a dead end. There was only so far I could go. The dead end appeared in the form of a 9 cm big fibroid in my uterus that was causing me to bleed heavily and become anemic. I not only had to turn around but also had to look deeply into what it meant to live with a uterus. And thus started my exploration.

MY JOURNEY WITH THE UTERUS

My journey started off in a naïve way. I first noticed that my abdomen was bulky. My immediate response was to ramp up my crunches and Pilates. If I had a tummy, it meant fat, right? Wrong. As I learnt, there are so many organs in the abdominal region that can bloat and bulk up due to reasons ranging from indigestion to periods. In my case an ultrasound revealed a big fibroid, a non-malignant tumour in the uterus. Fibroids occur in about thirty per cent women and are usually harmless except causing some discomfort during periods.

The medical professionals I consulted offered the most popular solution available in modern medicine – Hysterectomy. The process usually went like this:

I would be asked two questions.

1. How old are you?
2. Do you want to have more kids?

As I was forty and I was not planning on having more children, the solution was simple. "Get the uterus out. You don't need it. It has served its purpose."

In the western world, the prevalence of hysterectomy ranges from ten to twenty per cent among women in the latter half of the reproductive span. However, six in every hundred women aged thirty–forty-nine have had a hysterectomy in India. The prevalence is about eleven per one hundred women in the age group forty-five – forty-nine years.[1]

So, in this part of the world, hysterectomy was as common as getting a root canal.

I don't know what came over me. But I was determined that, if I was born with a uterus, I was going to die with one. I did not want to part with it halfway through my life.

My stubbornness made the doctors pause and give me the other alternate they knew. "Just wait," they said, "Menopause would shrink the fibroid." So, I just had to grow old, go through menopause and I will be fine. That sounded doable. Next step was to find out how much time I had. A girl likes to plan!

I asked my mum about the timing of her menopause. I learnt that she had had a hysterectomy, so she could not guide me on how the "tap" stopped.

"What about Grandma?"

"She had a hysterectomy too," my mum said.

What else could I expect in the land of hysterectomies? Seems like I could enter menopause in two years, or twelve years, I had no clue.

My mother however, broke the more popular myth that hysterectomy takes away the entire menopause experience. Apparently not. She went through a period of anxiety and irritation in her late fifties, corresponding to menopause. She confirmed that there is no escaping that. You may go under the knife, yet you have to suffer the period of being annoyed and reviewing the meaning of life (again!)

I was quite intrigued by how my conversations with women on menopause contrasted with the ones I had with men. I told my father I am researching on menopause. My father, a physician, said as a matter of fact, "Menopause is nothing. Your periods start coming at longer intervals. And after some time, it stops. That's all there is to it." My mom, listening to the conversation, took me aside and explained that it is a period of great anxiety and uncertainty. She was irritable all the time and could not quite understand what was going on. I wonder what my father thought of that phase. Or I. We neither cared to ask nor support her. Did we even know or notice that she was going through such a phase?

How can an inevitable phase of life for fifty per cent of the human population remain shrouded in such secret and misunderstanding? It was bewildering.

The answer, however, is not so hard to find. Women's bodies are hardly understood. We women, who carry them around don't know it ourselves. We are brave enough to stick our noses into a soiled diaper to check if it needs change, but do not try to understand the vagina, pubic bone, uterus, ovaries, cervix and how they all function. We buy a pack of sanitary pads every month, do whatever is needed to forget what we are going through and rush through life.

I remember pouring over the pages of a text by Margaret Sanger [2], my first foray into what a women's body was made of and how

---

2   *What every girl should know* by Margaret Sanger, first published in 1913

it worked. The real education however started later in life, in my forties when I switched to a menstrual cup, partly driven by being eco conscious and partly due to practicality; a standard napkin or a tampon could not absorb the outflow when I had my periods. Using a menstrual cup means no bars held. One must feel her way through the pubic bone into the cervix. I delivered two babies vaginally yet had no clue how my anatomy actually was until I started using the cup.

Around the same time, my crunches and tummy shaping underwear notwithstanding, I also started researching natural cures for my uterus – a long journey that took me through Yoga, Ayurveda, naturopathy and Tibetan practices.

ANCIENT PRACTICES

My exploration of menstrual health and menopause started with the system I am most familiar with, the modern allopathic medical system. My father and brother are both doctors. I grew up knowing basic medications, understanding medical terms and discussing medical procedures with the family. During the early part of my life, I truly believed that there is a pill for everything. Have a cold? Take an antibiotic. Antibiotic causes acidity? Take a Rantac.

It was a disappointment to discover that the magic of modern medicine was limited. Some of the deeper questions, especially with women's reproductive health remained unanswered.

For instance, when I was thirty-five, I chose to have my tubes tied. The doctor explained the procedure. The fallopian tubes will be scarred to stop the eggs from my ovaries reaching the uterus. It sounded like fixing a plumbing problem. Easy peasy! But the inquisitive me had a question. If the eggs don't reach the uterus, where exactly do they go? The doctor did not have a definite answer. Maybe it enters the blood stream, or maybe it disintegrates, she offered.

Fast forward, standing within perimenopause, and staring at menopause, my questions seem to have only increased.

At this point, almost all the women I have discussed menopause with had said two things:

1. Menopause hits parts of you that are already weak. People find that their chronic illnesses become enhanced during menopause. Dental issues crop up. (Dental and menopause? – I would not have made the connection in a thousand years!)
2. Menopause creates anxiety; a lot of it, sometimes leading to depression

Both these observations have led me to believe that the complications of menopause, more often than not are consequences of menstrual health during the previous years. Menstrual health on the other hand, is a consequence of one's lifestyle – the diet, the exercise, stress levels, sleep. The month-on-month menstruation deep cleans and resets a woman's body, flushing all toxins out. The process of menstruation is an indicator of how healthy a person has been in the month prior to the cycle.

As I started to research, I was not able to get very far with modern information that was available to me. So, I turned to Ayurveda. My first brush with Ayurveda was not much of a success and I ended up abandoning the treatment within a few months. That is the issue with treatment modalities like Ayurveda which are lifestyle based and highly individualised. Success arrives only when all things are aligned. My experience with Yoga and other modalities had worked really well before perimenopause. Perimenopause seemed like dull background in which everything you put in was getting lost. I had to look deeper.

Out of all the sastras, the sciences that I have learnt, Ayurveda offers the most comprehensive guide to this phase. In a crux, Ayurveda says this *'The entire period from menarche (onset of periods) to menopause is the journey of womanhood and this is celebrated. Woman's ability to bleed and reset makes her so powerful that she doesn't need many of the spiritual practices' men need to stay healthy and clear minded.'*

The texts prescribe knowledge and procedures around having healthy, and pain free cycles which have been lost. I grew up and continue to live in a society where discussing menstrual health and practices is considered embarrassing. For example, the neighbourhood pharmacist stores black plastic bags to wrap the pack every time I purchase sanitary napkins. He wouldn't be caught dead allowing a woman to carry her sanitary napkins out in the open! So, through my younger years I focused most of my energy on hiding the fact that I was on my moon cycle, rather than observing what was going on inside me. I have come a long way now making peace with the fact that I bleed and that it can stain. My younger self would find me abominable, a person incapable of leaving anything unstained when she has her periods! And worse, doesn't gush about it.

The very fact that menstrual cycles are to be enjoyed and celebrated is a notion I first came across in the novel, *The Red Tent*[2] based on the biblical character Dinah. The red tent was where women came together to bleed during their cycles every month. Their cycles were synchronised with the moon and with each other, and they bled during the new moon. A delightful passage from the book describes the first blood as the ripening of a woman. The women in the camp, sisters, mothers, aunts, handmaids, all gathered together in the "red tent" and sang songs that announced births, deaths and women's ripening to celebrate that. They rubbed henna on fingernails and soles of their feet. The girl who bled her first blood was adorned with every bangle, gem and jewel that could be found. The other women covered her head with the finest embroidery and sang songs for their Goddesses; for Inanna and Lady Asherah of the Sea, Elath and Anath, seeking their blessings.

It is similar to similar ceremonies that happen in my culture which we have been gradually moving away from. As a youngster I scorned at this ceremony and wished I did not have to go through it.

What does the ritual of the Red Tent or other similar rituals from around the world have to do with menopause? Many things. The more I learn and discover about ancient practices around periods and menopause, the more I decipher the depth of what we have lost.

We have lost the community. Most ancient traditions were designed to bring women together, every month for their moon cycle. The physical proximity and the emotional support and connection this provided extended through menopause, helping women navigate that phase of their lives with ease.

We have lost the connection with our bodies and this Earth and its cycles. We live in a world where our nights are lit up by electricity and schedules governed by deadlines. We are not in touch with our internal rhythms.

And we have lost celebrating the various stages of a woman's life, often fighting our bodies preferring to be stuck in bodies that look eighteen years of age. My culture has seven beautiful words for women in distinct stages of life. The interesting fact is that the stages are defined based on the cognitive and emotional maturity of the woman and not by age or looks. All ages were celebrated for what they brought to society. The current obsession with looking young and thin was not prevalent.

On the other side, we have also gained some. Women have a place and voice in the society and have a lot more agency in defining who we are and the choices we make in our lives. Our lives are not only about making babies.

As women living the years leading up to menopause, these are all factors to reflect upon and ones we can influence and change direction on. For, menopause can be hugely disruptive, destroying and creating at the same time.

AYURVEDA

I have to start with a disclaimer. There is a popular notion that everyone born in India practices Yoga every day and lives a life guided by Ayurvedic principles. The reality cannot be further from the truth. Yoga and Ayurveda are less understood in India than in many other parts of the world. We do have the advantage of access to age old knowledge written in language that we can follow and understand, but we don't have any other benefit of being born and lived here. I often feel like I straddle two worlds – my work in Technology and Diversity, Equity and Inclusion strongly placing me in a world of external achievements, leadership strategies, metrics and measures; when I return home and don the cape, I enter the world of Yoga and Ayurveda where experience matters more than numbers and reality is a question and not an absolute. The worlds remain divisively apart with a rare friend appearing in both.

What I am sharing here is from the view of a learner and a practitioner, finding my way through the maze, not as an expert.

Ayurveda is an ancient medical system that originated in India. The difference that sets Ayurveda apart from most other healing systems is that Ayurveda emphasises on daily lifestyle than just stepping in when things are not right. Maintaining homeostasis is a better strategy than treating illness. As Dr. Robert Svoboda confirms, "Ayurveda is a renowned medical system, but medicine is a small portion of the voluminous tapestry of its knowledge."

To further clarify, the experience I share here is also based on lifestyle learnings from Ayurveda and not the medical part of it.

INTRODUCTION TO AYURVEDA

According to Ayurveda, a human body is a combination of three doshas or principles, Vata, Pitta and Kapha. These three are condensed forms of the five natural elements this world is made of: Earth, Fire, Water, Air and Space. You will find references to the five elements in the Chinese medicine and Feng shui as well, with Wood and Metal replacing the Space and Air elements.

A simple meditation

For a few minutes, I would like you to forget about anatomy, the different body systems and all other parts and workings of the body we learnt in the science class at school. Let us do a small experiment. Sit comfortably in a place where you are not likely to be disturbed for at least five minutes. Bring your attention and awareness to where you are sitting, how you are resting on the seat. Roll your shoulders back and down. Close your eyes. Exhale, just letting it all out. Bring your awareness to your body, this place we live in during our time on Earth.

Bring your awareness back to your seat, and how your sitting bones to meet the cushion or the mat. Allow your weight to sink in. Do you get a sense of the Earth as you find the seat holding you and your body settling into it?

From here, take your awareness into the rest of your body, especially to your blood vessels. Can you get a sense of blood flowing through your vessels? The cells of your body are filled with seventy per cent water. Feel it brimming and flowing through your body.

Gently bring your attention to your abdomen, your navel to be exact. Stay there for a few breaths to see if you can become aware of the warmth in your belly. It's the Fire. The digestive fire and the fire of your energy resides there. Chinese healing arts call it the Qi. Stay with the Fire.

Now, move your awareness to your breath. For the next few breaths, greet every inhalation like you would welcome a friend coming home. Follow the breath through your nose, throat and the chest and deeper if you can. Become aware of the Air element as your body expands on inhalation and rests on exhalation.

With the next exhalation, follow the breath until you reach a point where nothing remains. Surrender to that stillness. That is your experience of the Space element. Where can you feel it around you, in you?

Now gently come back, move your head and neck slowly and once you feel ready, open your eyes.

You have just had an experience of the five elements. Unlike modern medicine where I can show you the photographs of the heart or ultrasound of the abdomen, the eastern medicine can only be explained and understood energetically.

The Three Doshas

For the sake of understanding and working with human physiology, Ayurveda condenses the above five elements into three doshas.

Vata is the kinetic energy of the body. This is influenced by the Air element and is responsible for all movements by the body and within the body.

Kapha is the potential energy of the body. It lubricates, maintains and protects the body. It is the stabilising influence, in a sense the opposite of Vata. Think blood, mucus and other fluids in the body when you think Kapha. Kapha is influenced by the Water element. I also find that Kapha relates to the Earth element, stabilising and holding me.

Pitta is the fire that pushes one to move forward and grow. Thus, Pitta is the transformational energy. It controls the balance of Vata and Kapha and is majorly influenced by the Fire element. I have experienced Pitta to also have qualities of the Space element allowing a human being to expand and create.

Ayurveda's primary objective is to keep the three doshas in balance. It is very rare to find human beings who have all the doshas in balance. Most people have two dominating doshas and some have one dominating dosha. Like all things in life, anything in excess is not a good thing. There are plenty of resources online where you can check which doshas are predominant in your constitution, although it is best to work with someone who is practicing Ayurvedic healing.

Here's the other thing. The knowledge of the three doshas doesn't slot you conveniently into a bucket, like the twelve sun signs (I always wondered if 1/12th of the entire world ended up with the same luck as mine!) or even the personality types of MBTI (Myers-Brigg Type Indicator). The doshas are influenced by the time of the day, the season of the year, the place one lives in and one's age. So, it is fluid and very unique to every person.

Women's life stage and dominant doshas

Let us look at a slice of this relationship between doshas and all other factors which matters to us.

Women's life can be roughly divided into three stages – Childhood, Womanhood and the Wise Age[3]. I am taking these as broad classifications. The individual circumstances may vary.

Childhood is the time between birth and adulthood, the growth phase. During this phase, the girl child has a dominant Kapha. This is the phase that sets the ground for future personality, life choices and attitude. So, it is natural that Kapha leads, creating a stable ground. When you consider that the baby swims in the womb when she is a fetus and that she lives on a liquid diet through her infancy the water/fluid nature of Kapha makes more sense. Among the different tastes, sweet is attributed to Kapha, so it is not surprising that children are sweet, and they have a sweet tooth.

Womanhood is the period between, probably eighteen and up to the late forties. This is the time when the woman in menstruating, is likely to have children and invest herself in her career and life aspirations. The dominant dosha during this period is Pitta, bringing with it the fire like ambition and intent to grow and achieve. Many of us turn perfectionists during this case, becoming highly sensitive to criticism and negative feedback. Most of the lifestyle diseases take root during this phase.

Wise woman is the stage from menopause into other decades. Women live longer than men and it is not unusual for us to look forward to spending 3 to 4 decades in this phase. This delightful wisdom phase, where we let go off worrying about others and have a chance to enjoy the pleasures of life is dominated by Vata, the air element. Like air, this is the time to disseminate what you have learnt and experienced in your life.

We don't have a term for the transition from childhood to womanhood. Adolescence and teenage comes close. But the intense psychological stress I felt as I tore myself away from the comfort of home to discover myself as an individual was quite significant. It caused me to falter and take flawed decisions. But that phase was not marked by physical changes.

The second transition, as we move from Womanhood to Wise woman, comes with physical indicators which makes this transition a lot harder than the previous one. But it is only a transition and an inevitable phase of life.

As I was researching for this piece, I discovered an interesting fact. No other non-human primates go through menopause. There is current research emerging that Beluga whales go through menopause, but on the land, this seems to a unique human experience. And that made me wonder, why on earth did I sign up for being a female human? Dr. Jared Diamond thinks this is an evolutionary tactic. The older a woman gets, the riskier it becomes for her to become pregnant and rear children. We would rather have fewer surviving children whom we had a chance to raise right, with proper nutrition and care than a vast number of children. As a social species, we probably also made this choice to enable older women to help with delivery and baby care of other women. I guess our ancestors didn't quite take into account that women one day would turn the long years with no periods or young children to care for, into a vacation.

Vata, The Mischief Maker

Without going into too many details, let me just say this. When it comes to period flow and menopause, Vata is the chief disturbance officer. Pitta and Kapha do play a role (think hot flashes and weight gain), but this is primarily a Vata show. I might be simplifying this, but unless you are planning on diving deep into Ayurveda, this is a good base for us to move forward with.

What exactly is Vata?

"There are twenty-five browser tabs open on my laptop and I don't know where the music is coming from." Sound familiar, or even feel familiar? This is Vata, a force that pushes you to move towards things. Distractions, restlessness, the go-go-go attitude, Fear of missing out (FOMO) are all expressions of Vata. I could be defining an entire generation here, but my life was exactly like this. Vata is the predominant force required to make the blood flow. A disturbance to Vata, too much of it or too less of it is bound to cause cramps and other issues.

Menopause brings the next layer of complication. With menopause, we move into a Vata dominant phase. So, while the Vata that pushes the menstrual blood out is increasing in the body, your body is trying to stop producing ovaries and get off the wagon. There is a force that aids your menstrual flow, and the same force is also working to stop the process altogether. Talk about getting communication lines mixed up!

However, Ayurveda doesn't see menopause as a period of confusion. This phase is considered a period of rebirth. Women are prescribed various fats, in the form of oils and ghee (clarified butter) made from cow's ghee for consumption and applying on the bodies, especially joints. Women are asked to take care of themselves like a newborn baby, surrounding themselves with loving and supportive people to help transition through. It is as joyous a journey as coming into adolescence but lacks the support it needs.

AND SO IT ALL BEGAN

When I started my journey, I didn't quite know all this. It has taken me four years to start tying the pieces together.

A clip I watched from the television series Fleabag (Prime video) summarises my learnings delightfully. It has Kirsten Scott-Thomas, in her flawless style of delivery, talking about how women are born with pain built-in. Periods, child birth, sore boobs, breasts overflowing with milk, all of these bring pain and women live with them. Men on the other hand, have to seek it out by creating Gods and demons and wars. When they don't have wars, they play rugby. They do that so that they can feel, touch each other and feel pain and guilt. Women do it very well on their own aided by periods. Just when women think they have made peace with periods and emotions, menopause hits, crumbling the pelvic floor and making one hot and old at the same time. But after that intense period, woman is free!

I wasn't quite thinking menopause when I started seeking help for my fibroid. Menopause as I came to discover, isn't a singular event that happens in a woman's late forties. It is a process that sets in between thirty – thirty-five years. The emotional upheavals, the food habits, the work stress, the physical health all start charting the path one's menopause would take. Nobody tells you that. And we spend those years trying to get pregnant, losing sleep over young kids or traveling furiously around the world for work – none of which need to be stopped, but to be worked on with balance and awareness.

My first indication that something could be wrong was my annual ultrasound. The sonologist chatted with me about my fibroid. "You have a fibroid."

"Uh hum" – I had no clue what that meant.

"Do you have heavy bleeding?"

"No" – I didn't, at the time.

"You can go for a hysterectomy if you like. But it looks ok for now."

This exchange repeated for a few years. I came away with a smirk every year wondering at the suggestion of hysterectomy. Until - until the bleeding did become an issue.

On my personal side my marriage was going through a stressful phase. I had started a technology company and my venture wasn't doing too well adding financial strain. I simply wasn't connecting the dots. My menstrual health, which had usually been too insignificant to give any mind space, was beginning to become a pivotal point of my life. I was stopped at airports and asked if I was pregnant. It was embarrassing.

My first step was to work with my diet. I noticed that some foods, especially processed foods increased my bloating and blood flow. I had to cut those out. I am quite fortunate that God gave me stoic taste buds, compensating for a bleeding heart. I could give up foods quite easily. Our generation's obsession with thin bodies only helped. If a food would make me fat, I wouldn't eat it; now if a food would make me bleed, I was going to cut it out. I experimented and started avoiding foods that seemed to increase the blood flow. I gave up most processed food and some spices like fenugreek and chilies. I limited my sweets. And all that seemed to help. A bit, but after time things went back to being heavy. My bloating increased, especially before my cycle, bringing up with its acidity.

This is when I decided to try Ayurveda - my first attempt, which did not go so well. I was prescribed a set of ghritas (medicated ghee). I went with that for about 6 months during which things did not change much.

All through this phase, the suggestions for hysterectomy did not cease. Having failed in my attempt with Ayurveda, I turned to modern medicine. I did my research and consulted the top gynecologist in town. I requested for a myomectomy, which involved only removing the bulky fibroid but leaving my uterus intact. As I prepared for the surgery, I discovered a few things that made me question my decision. For one, this was going to be an open surgery which meant I would need three - six months of recovery time. Second, the doctor could not guarantee that the surgery will cure my excessive bleeding, or she would actually be able to save my uterus, both my very purposes of going into surgery. The week before I went in, India announced lockdowns for COVID. I never called the hospital back to reschedule my surgery.

Third attempt is usually lucky. The third attempt stresses me out when I am dealing with passwords, but in other places it is often lucky. A friend spoke highly of a naturopath, and I decided to check this option out. Mr. Moorthy is an interesting healer, who will only meet you in person, alone, in his dimly lit office. The pandemic was not a reason enough for him to tele/ video consult; in fact, he did not own a smartphone. His methods were equally different from anything else one would come across. There were some herbal remedies involved, but it mostly consisted of lifestyle changes, peculiar diets and prescriptive showers. At that point, I did not quite understand why he was asking me to make those changes, but it all makes sense now.

The first step was to cut down on my activity level. At this point, I was running, hiking, learning Kalari (a South Indian martial art form), practicing Yoga, lifting weights and had a consistent practice of Tibetan rites. It may not sound like much to some of you but hear me out. I was constantly adding more activities to my life. Every one of this was aggravating my Vata. Every movement, of the mind or the body, was increasing my Vata, which was not being balanced enough. This high Vata was most likely contributing to the heavy bleeding.

We live in a world where achievement is highly rated. The ability to multi-task and in general, do more is a desirable quality. I especially have been admired for finding the energy and time to do "so many things." To cut back on activities that I loved to do was really, really hard. I felt useless and incapable.

The second part was the diet. This shouldn't be hard, or so I thought. But the healing diet he prescribed was devoid of all fermented food, lemon, chilies, coffee, wine, garlic, ginger, nuts and chocolate. If you don't know people from my part of the world, the southern part of India, you may not grasp how difficult such a diet is. The chief breakfast of the region is idli, a fermented steamed preparation made of rice and black lentils. You cannot find any dish here that is devoid of chilies. Adding chocolates, coffee and wine to the mix was horrendous. As I went on this diet, I lost weight the first couple of months and almost fainted when I went on a hike. I simply did not know what to eat that did not involve fermented food or chilies. This also came in the way of cutting down of my already non-existent social life. "Six months, Maggie," I told myself. That's all I was going to give this crazy path.

The third was to eliminate cosmetics and make up. This was a hard shift as well. While I am not a heavy make-up user, giving up on the basics threatened to make a dent on my self-esteem. Ah well, what is self-esteem with a bulky abdomen? I braved this one as well.

As the days went, things changed. Quite significantly, in fact. My skin cleared up and brightened. My bleeding reduced. My haemoglobin levels came back up to double digits after hovering dangerously in single digits for years. My therapist's message was consistent. "It is time you focus on yourself."

Coming back to Ayurveda

During this phase, my Yoga practice also changed significantly. The school where I learn Yoga focuses more on the breath than acrobatics. As I turned my attention to breath, I observed that my exhalations were short and labored. This is one more malady of our modern times. We are in such a rush to consume and are so insecure by what we cleverly call the VUCA world, that we cannot let go. This manifests as short and laboured outbreath.

At a more subtle level this is an indicator of Apana Vayu not working effectively. Who is this new friend, Apana? Vata has five sub-doshas – Prana, Apana, Samana, Udana and Vyana. These refer to the directions of movement in various systems of the body. Apana is especially related to the elimination function of the body. An imbalance of this Vayu (roughly translates to energy flow) leads to menstrual issues (could also cause constipation, diarrhea, overactive bladder etc.)

As I started the long and disciplined work with the breath, I started noticing a few things with my menstrual cycle:

- My diet and emotional health directly reflected on how much my abdomen bloated that month and how stressful my cycle was that month.
- It helped not to do strenuous physical activities during the first two days of my period.
- Estrogen in general increased by abdomen bloating and bleeding. And estrogen got in through many sources – natural foods like soy, over exercising and cosmetics. Most shampoos and creams contain estrogen. Estrogen in turn increases the size of the fibroid. The lesser the cosmetics, lower the estrogen getting into my body.

My seventy-five-year-old Yoga teacher is an expert in women's health. After working with me for six months, she suggested I see an Ayurveda doctor and get some medications in. I was hesitant to go through the same phase again, but it has been a refreshing experience aided by my current knowledge and experience in working with myself. I currently take some herbs, continue to stay on a restricted diet that soothes the Vata and continue to work with my breath. Has my fibroid disappeared yet? Not yet. My abdomen seems to have shrunk a tiny bit, but I really don't care. I feel a lot better; my energy has improved, and health indicators are looking good. I have learnt to see my body as the moon, waxing and waning with cycles, and not be hung up about a certain body shape. All I needed was a bigger wardrobe with more choices. I look at the coming years as a preparation towards menopause and a transition to the wise woman phase without shaking my world too much. Because you know, I have work to do and people to love.

A NOTE ON ESTROGEN

The estrogen connection with women's menstrual health interestingly, is lesser known, especially with regards to menopause because women's bodies are supposed to produce less estrogen as we near menopause. In his book *What the doctor may not tell you about menopause* Dr. John Lee introduces the term "estrogen dominance." Many women in their mid-thirties begin to have cycles where they do not ovulate. This results in their bodies producing less progesterone while the levels of estrogen remain the same. This is what Dr. John Lee terms as estrogen dominance. He associates a number of symptoms from weight gain, heavy and irregular bleeding, mood swings and hair loss to this condition.

The natural cycles apart, we also are prone to absorbing estrogen from other sources. How does extra estrogen get into our bodies? Dr. Ananya Mandal suggests we look for the below terms on the labels of cosmetics you buy –

- Parabens – These are used extensively as a preservative in low amounts (0.1-0.3 per cent by weight per ingredient). Types include butylparaben, ethyl paraben, isobutyl paraben, methylparaben, propylparaben.

- Placental Extracts – these contain hormones estrogen, estrone, and progesterone as contaminants. They are found in shampoos, conditioners, moisturisers and astringents, body and skin creams.

- UV Screens – these are UV protection creams and photo-stabilisers. They are used in considerable amounts of two-fifteen per cent by weight per ingredient. Many commonly used UV-screens are absorbed by the skin and get access to the blood stream. They are found in sunscreens, perfumes, hair sprays, shampoos, conditioners, styling gels, facial creams, foundations, moisturisers, lipsticks, liquid hand soaps, body wash, insect repellants, nail polish and polish remover, and aftershave and shaving creams. The harmful chemicals in UV screens are benzophenone-1, benzophenone-2, homosalate, octinoxate, oxybenzone, sulisobenzone, and 4-MBC (this is used in Europe but not in the United States).

THE THIRTIES, THE PERIMENOPAUSE AND THE PATH TO MENOPAUSE

As my journey continues, I shake my head at the comments we used to make about our periods. "Why do women have this?" "Won't this bloody thing just stop?" Let me tell you two things, my dear young women at the prime of your age –

1. There is no real "prime of your age," it is a shifting goal post. It actually gets better.
2. When you get to the point where it is going to stop, you are more likely to wish for it go on, for some more time

Let me not paint a false picture. Vata increases as you hit menopause because your body begins to "dry out" in some sense. Your skin starts to wrinkle, the joints begin to lose their lubrication and hair starts to fall. But the knowledge of this does not have to turn you away from the inevitable. Think Jane Fonda, Jane Goodall, Pema Chodron. Here is your chance to grow into your own gleaming, glistening sparkle of a wise woman; Bhairavi as Vedic traditions would call her.

The fantastic thing is that you have the key right with you – your current menstrual health.

Here are some indicators. If your flow is scanty with a lot of cramps, your Vata is high. If you are missing your period because of hectic travel schedule or activity, that is also an indicator of high Vata. A heavy, hot flow and an irritable mood may point to a high Pitta. Increased water retention and depression tells you that your Kapha is out of balance. Again, this is at an elevated level. You will need to work with a practitioner to understand your body type clearly and how you can balance a dosha.

However, you can take charge, slow down if your periods tell you to, move to the right diet and take care of your emotional and mental health. It is never too early to start investing in this part of you.

This investment comes with also building or tapping into a kind and compassionate community. We have long derided groups of women coming together to laugh and share food. "I do not like to gossip" has been a proud statement of many of us, women achievers. Make your own circle that shares your passion, interests and definitely, food, a vegan granola circle, if that's what works. But women thrive and flourish when we come together. Solitude doesn't abode well for most of us. Find your sisterhood, exchange stories and walk together.

In a world that glorifies youth and loud, vocal achievements, be the quiet revolution who shines her light on others, just by being her best self.

Put menopause on the map. Seriously.

REFERENCES:

Shekhar, C., Paswan, B. & Singh, A. Prevalence, sociodemographic determinants and self-reported reasons for hysterectomy in India. *Reprod Health* **16,** 118 (2019).

Ayurveda for Women – A Guide to Vitality and Health, Dr Robert E. Svoboda

Reflections

Reflections

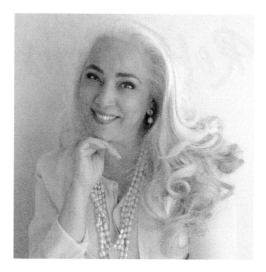

LIANA CHAOULI
USA

Liana Chaouli, (pronounced sha-oo-li), is the President and Founder of Image Therapists International Inc. and a globally recognised thought leader, S.T.Y.L.E. Sage™ educator and innovator.

Ms. Chaouli, best-selling author of "You Are a Masterpiece," provides transformation through the empowerment of language, wardrobe and self-beliefs. She has spent over 4 decades consulting CEOs, celebrities, and political figures on matters of self-image.

As the developer of Image Therapy™, she works closely with her clients on their personal and professional presence using analysis, physical appearance, and education to adjust attitudes affecting self-esteem and overall sense of worth. Her clients include US Bank, Bob Mackie, The Canfield Training Group (Jack Canfield, Chicken Soup for the Soul), KTLA (Los Angeles), IBM, Nordstrom's, Department of Defence, Harvard and The Home Base Foundation, Coldwell Banker University, Chico's, and many more.

To find out how to work with Liana, please visit https://imagetherapists.com

Chapter Ten

ME NO PAUSE... I WILL NOT PAUSE MY LIFE FOR IT

"I woke up the other morning and realised I missed you. To anyone listening to me as I spoke with you in my moments of sadness, they would think I was talking to a lover or a dear friend, and in some ways they would be right. You have been a dear friend, and one I never fully appreciated until it was too late."

It was early on a cold Sunday morning when this very loud feeling, this conversation woke me up, not just on a physical level but also on a deep soul level. It was more like a craving, an emptiness, like the longing we have to reconnect with a close friend whom we have not hugged for many years.

Sitting up in my warm bed, surrounded by the wonderful memories of a life lived, I whispered "I miss you" into the darkness of my beautiful boudoir.

I spoke as though my utterance could lighten these moments of lack. As my words filled the room, tears fell gently like those of a child. The loud voice reverberating in my brain matched the beating at the base of my heart, both of which pulled me into this unexpected moment; and it was shocking.

Anyone listening would have sworn that my emotional entrance into this awakening was on account of a lover, a person whom I was close to, a good man who had gotten away or even just the loss of a deep connection.

It wasn't a lover, or a friend, but a deep connection with another person, the person within me, the woman I used to be.

"I miss you" I whispered. And as my ears and my soul heard these words from my own voice, I knew this awakening was a letting go; an embrace of love for the woman I have become and am becoming.

I miss my periods. I miss the cycle. I miss knowing that I can create life inside this beautiful, soft and strong body of mine. I miss the monthly reminder of womanhood. I miss my soul's tenderness a few days before, during and after. I miss the scent, the texture, the fear of sitting on white chairs, the unknown tears, all the ups and down, all the cramps, the excuses, all of it.

I just miss the feeling of being a woman in that way.

In this tender moment, all the pain, all the resentment I felt for myself and for this "curse" we had to endure as girls, showed up. And to my shock it presented itself as mourning rather than anger.

In a split second my heart went from hate to gratitude, and I longed to feel all of those feelings again, all the markings which were my path to maturity.

Every ruby drop had made me who I am today, and after years of resenting, berating and rejecting, I now felt blessed with love, grace and gratitude for every drop.

For it is these rich drops, these raw and powerful emotions we women experience, all the fears and all the shame instilled within us over centuries of challenges, which have made us who we are today.

It is this new awareness of who we are, this 'IT' rising within us which has ushered global communities of women to awaken and unleash their womanhood. We are waking up and experiencing life at a whole new level as we enter this powerful time of transformation, a time which I am eternally grateful for.

Looking back on this beautiful journey, which every girl and woman will experience in her own individual, often clumsy way, I remember the abrupt traumatic experience my mother put me through at the tender age of ten.

Allow me to invite you into this moment and share a little bit of the shock I felt the ten-year-old Lilli. The little girl that I was, who together with my sister was doing homework in our shared bedroom, turned around to look up at our mother as she entered our room. I quickly started fretting with anxiety and an impending sense of shame.

I knew and felt as though I had done something wrong. The room was charged with blame, tension, rather than beautiful tenderness. The lack of kindness and empathy burned this moment into my soul, joining the basket of traumatic childhood experiences.

Let's be clear, what unfolded was caused by unspoken fears emanating from both my mother and myself, unspoken fears passed down from generation to generation.

My mother's concern for my well-being after discovering my smudged panties tucked away, hidden at the bottom of the dirty laundry hamper, was a fear she never communicated to me. This wasn't just a moment of 'Oh, she got her period' this was the beginning of me being able to get pregnant, of becoming a woman in my own right.

For the mother of a young Persian Jewish girl, this was a time of letting go of her daughter's innocence, letting go of my safety, of my childhood, all wrapped up in fears I had no knowledge of. This was a time of protection: protecting me, protecting the family, protecting the purity of our culture and faith. I was no longer allowed to visit friends at home, play after school or stay with friends on the weekend.

And then there was my fear: fear of what was happening down there, being fearful of the unknown, fearful of my mother's wrath inherited through generations of needing to be strong and resilient women.

As my mother charged in the room, coupled with my feelings of having done something wrong increasing and rising within me, my mother told me to pull down my panties. She wanted to see the smudging, and as I obeyed this request, all the feelings of guilt and shame took residence on levels I wouldn't truly understand until my later years.

My mother then took me outside into the back garden, urged me to scream at the top of my lungs into the vastness of the sky above, without explanation, without tenderness, and without reassurance of what was to come. Just in a straightforward 'let's get it done' way, typical of my mother.

Not communicating fears with each other as mother and daughter wasn't unique to us. It was the story of mothers and daughters the world over, of sisters and of friends. This 'IT' had created a communication breakdown between females of all ages.

There was no forewarning to the smudging or this traumatic experience with my mother in the garden. There was just this 'heed the fear of getting the curse' experience. No explanation, just a doing which set the tone of my periods, before working its way through my life and eventually my menopause in a way that is so beautifully profound in the rawness of it all.

This is the kind of experience that so many of us little girls lived through, in one way or another. Getting our period was a curse! The truth is, or rather MY truth is: when my cycle hit me, it hit me early, I was still a child who was in no way prepared for any of IT.

No one had prepared me for the fact that something was going to happen to me, nor that my undies were to suddenly show signs of the smudging, something that didn't even look like blood. The first time a young girl gets her period it's not usually the rivers of red, which we often associate with bleeding, no, it's just a trickle…and it's a dry brown trickle. It's not the look of blood, it doesn't resemble anything you know, and this made it scary. I had no idea what was happening to me, I was so afraid, deeply ashamed of the unknown thing that was happening to me, down there, in my undies.

To add insult to injury amongst this fear and confusion, my mother gets me to do this crazy, absolutely absurd ritual which traumatised me on a deep level. Years later I understood that it was this experience which led to many years of painful periods. Every month I would be doubled up in pain, lying in my bed crying, the tears a mix of pain and fear, mostly feeling as though I had somehow done something wrong, like it was some kind of punishment handed down to me by God.

No one tells you when you are five years old that your life will be thwarted into the beginning of your future, by the periods, the emotions, and this untapped life-giving power, nor do they tell you there is an ending to them, which needs a ceremony, a reverence, with grace, welcoming in the book ending of our lives.

My mother didn't tell me until years later that this screaming at the top of my voice, into the vastness of space around me, had a beautiful and empowering message at the heart of it. That with the smudging came the gift of being a woman, a woman who had a voice to use, and use it I must. This was in direct contradiction to the lack of voice so many women around me, and around the world had and still have.

This magnificent message of using my voice, and the gift of womanhood is not shared with us like a wonderful fairy tale or soothing bedtime story when we need it the most. As a little girl starting to grow up, looking up to her "elders," sisters, mum, aunties or friends this lack of knowledge, this lack of shared experience, the lack of feminine intimacy with the women who mattered most to me in my life, left me wondering why no one spoke of what was to come.

I could have never imagined the ways in which this 'IT' would change my young life in the ways it then did. Getting my period, without warning, and with no awareness or mention of this thing that would inevitably happen to me, happen for me, was a journey I was meant to walk alone. I was meant to discover profound yet painful things my own way, and though that may seem wonderful now, at the time it was one of the most painful experiences of my then short life.

My mother wasn't trying to be cruel, far from it. She was loving and smart, beautiful inside and out, but the monthly debilitating pain was the exact opposite.

You may not think that menopause, the very idea of it, the way we live or shy away from "the CHANGE," couldn't possibly start when you're a very young girl. How could it? As a free spirit sailing on playground swings while devouring your favourite chocolate ice cream, you're not thinking of life in your fifties or sixties. You are there in the moment flying through life free as a bird with the deliciousness of chocolate in the corners of your mouth.

But it is in this moment something happens, and you gain access to an inner knowing of something stirring deep inside of you. You can't name it, you can't even describe it, but your soul knows. My soul knew. It was this this knowing that carried me through the later years of my periods to my point of no return, MY menopause.

Being a young Jewish girl of Persian ancestry, raised in Europe, a polyglot, learning, living and speaking the languages of Farsi, Italian, French, English, Hebrew and Yiddish which surrounded me as I grew up, was an extraordinary experience. These multicultural influences from my diverse family and social circles left me confused, pulled into so many different cultural norms.

Being Jewish I was raised with the beliefs that during the time of our cycle, we as women are not clean, even though I washed every morning and night, tried to behave myself and believed in the Divine. How could I not be clean?

This belief of being unclean was further enforced by my grandmother who told me I was not even allowed to make yoghurt with her when the bleeding came.

As the years went by no one said to me "Come let me show what this will be like, let me give you a taste of the diversity of what could happen, and here is a safe place where you can bring your concerns or ask any of your questions." No one told me the power of the period, or the magnificence of menopause. In fact, no one in my family, or social circles ever spoke about any of 'IT' – this forbidden subject of womanhood.

I honestly do not remember any woman in my family ever speaking about 'IT'. My grandmother lived with us for most of the latter part of her life, never did I hear her mention 'IT'. My mother, who's eighteen years older than me, and should by all accounts have had 'IT' when I was around thirty-six or so, never ever mentioned 'IT'.

'IT' was not an open part of their lives. My many aunties, eight to be exact: three female powerhouses on my mum's side and five strong matriarchs on my dad's, were not a source of personal female education either. They were the next closest female role models I could have looked towards, yet they lived so far away in distance as well as their ability to support. Not that they were purposely withholding, I feel their path was not guided by grace either, so they just lived this 'IT-ness' as they were shown by women who came before them.

The one aunty I cherished, loved and felt closest to was my mother's older sister Sheherazad. She was a soldier, an opera singer, an artist proficient in ten languages including Latin, Arabic, Greek and Russian just to name a few, overall she was a Shaman of the utmost excellence. And even she never spoke about IT, at least not in my presence.

As I grew older, more cultural influences were painted into my life. I soon began to realise the messages women are fed about our bodies, about our journeys, and about some of those most important things which happen for us in life.

The German influence fed me the narrative that this phase of our lives, our monthly cycle – our periods - are completely normal. We're not unclean, we just need to be clean - check for leakages, keeping sanitary items with us at all times. Just in case. Very pragmatic.

My Persian background held a similar narrative to being Jewish. This 'IT,' the combination of periods and menopause, is never to be talked about in public, or with members of the opposite sex. We were unclean, had to be clean and were to sleep apart from our husbands when in this state of uncleanliness.

The Italian influence fed me a similar narrative to the German. It was a softer, more sensual massage, one with more accepting focus towards our internal selves, our bodies, our powerfulness, our womanness and motherhood.

Embracing all of these influences over the years I feel blessed because I had a wide expanse of knowledge and culture many women or young girls do not have access to. This richness of diversity of cultural wisdom is hidden from them, like it was for me in my younger years.

As I'm writing this, immersing myself in thoughts, engaging with my own experience of menopause, I think about the fact that there is no university.

There's no place where we as women can go to learn about our bodies, our sensuality, our sexuality. Why do we not offer a 'period' class in school? We are expected to learn skills, educated ourselves through science, languages and geography, yet there is no "Teenage ~ social awkwardness ~ body rollercoaster" class. There's English, history, trigonometry, and of course there's geometry, yet there's barely anything that teaches girls what to do when they get their period and for most of us, we don't get it at home either. Like I said … we need a "Teenage ~ social awkwardness ~ body function ~ understanding ~ emotional rollercoaster" class, for young boys as well as girls!

Many of us didn't have mothers, sisters, or aunts who talked to us about 'IT'. My grandmother sure as hell didn't talk about it, IT wasn't the thing to do.' I haven't met anyone who's actually had a grandmother, mother, aunt, older sisters or cousin who sat them down and said, "You know what sweetheart, here's what's going to happen to you: in the next few years, this will be part of your life. As you grow up, slowly becoming a woman, maturing into womanhood, these are the things you are going to encounter." Nothing and no-one. Period. Why was I schooled in how to be a good wife, but not on how to be a woman? A sensual, sexual and divine woman? A woman who leads herself and others with compassion, love and radical self-acceptance. One who shows up wearing her tender vulnerabilities, her femininity and deliciousness like a majestic crown, as she includes others less able to boldly forge ahead in togetherness. Our Sensuality is sacred, it is a much-needed super ingredient for LIFE itself.

There is no sensuality university, there is no femininity university, there is no college that curates all the information that we need as women to empower us on this forever winding path.

This mysteriously vast world of being a woman doesn't have an all-knowing professor we can question. There is no "Hogwarts " boarding school which we can attend or go to meet other women. A safe human home where we can share ideas, learn from our elders as we are experiencing life in the moment. A sanctuary where we are being loved, nurtured and supported by them. Because it is not available It doesn't exist… YET I see a sacred space, life sanctuary, an educational encounter for any stage of this beautifully intricate tapestry of feminine living. Call it what you like, we need to build it for the sake of our children. For the sake of their empowerment as they learn to live life from a generous space of peaceful self-acceptance.

We make our way through life in a state of not knowing, in pain, in fear and we rely on pieces of information given to us here and there, all wrapped up in the unkindness of disgust, embarrassment and the fear of being discovered. A narrative of our journey is distorted by time, by what has history taught us about our bodies, by men and women alike.

Women were not allowed to be doctors, we were not allowed to speak, not allowed to engage in conversations, not only with men, but with each other. There was no empowerment such as what we have and are developing today.

My future was to be a wife. That was my path, especially since it was the only way to leave home. Marriage was the answer to my yearning for my independence. Little did I know that is choosing one sort of confinement for yet another. I remember the way I had been schooled on how to be a good wife, how as a woman I would need to sleep in a separate bed from my husband every month. This was to protect HIM from my lack of cleanliness, to prevent his embarrassment and discomfort. These quietly hushed conversations further deepened the feelings of shame. They reinforced my "being dirty". With every month of my red rivers, the arrival of more guilt and embarrassment for being a woman arose within me.

We were not allowed to discuss or question our journey, not in society, in religion, or in the supposedly sacred realm of the family. No one ushers us through it, because no one ushered our mothers, aunties and grandmothers through it. This is where the forgiveness of these beautiful women in our lives comes to the fore. Where we start the healing process of the pain. We can choose to transcend the traumas of our bodies. With compassionate willingness we will sooth our scared souls, as we tend to them in loving grace.

Our female hearts, the feminine journey is as diverse as the grains of sand on the beach. So… I ask you, how could there ever have been a faculty of knowing, when the women before us didn't discuss their experiences? How could they have known when this knowledge, the listening to and the honouring of our bodies was stolen from them and us by a mandate of silence? Today looking at this wonderful place via hindsight, I see that the awakening of an understanding of this transformation of mine, this 'IT' no one spoke of, did start in the moments of screaming up to the sky, of being the free spirit on the swing, the curious child wondering at the goings on in my own body.

This 'IT', this passage we all must live through and with, starts in our childhood. IT starts with our very own tribe which embraces or abhors this THING. We are either blessed or cursed with the open minds of those who came before us, their ability or willingness to share this "What's about to happen to you journey". Some of us are lucky enough to actually be guided by angel mothers, whose wisdom envelopes our life with endless compassion for our woman walk.

But not all of us, not me, and possibly not you.

Some of us think we are doing it wrong, and we don't know how to handle this thing, this 'IT', so we become masculine trying to run from it. Some of us become a man either by shifting our physical self or by emulating men in the way we do business, in the way we dress or the way we live. We resist the change, and then suddenly, before we know it, 'IT' comes along, our cycle, our vibrancy and fertility get stolen by an unseen thief in the night.

Those of us who stay the course, we find ourselves with rivers of the Amazon running down our bodies. These physical expressions which challenge and confront us without the planning, without the preparation. These moments of embarrassment which show up in the most inconvenient times are also the best of times because they are real. This change in us is real. 'IT' is powerful and it is Divinely given to us as a gift of awakening into the wise woman we truly are. I believe we can give this wisdom to others, to our daughters, our nieces, and to our men. Yes, our men, our sons and nephews, our male colleagues and friends. This is a gift we can no longer keep to ourselves once we have understood the powerful lusciousness of it all.

IT becomes a dance we are invited to at any given moment. We can either accept or decline the invitation. When we choose to accept IT, we are accepting a dance into the unknown world of our ultimate power, laced with a fire of vast proportions which depend on who we are and who we choose to become. We may not realise it at the time, but we are also accepting the opportunity to embrace who we really are. This can be the portal which leads to graceful self-acceptance of the Centurion Woman inside all of us.

Yes! YOU A Centurion Woman! Each of us leading hundreds of other women with reverence and resilience. We help them rise with courage, confidence, a strength and most importantly with the tender sensuality which commands attention.

I now know I was perimenopausal when the nightly hot flashes visited me, making me restless. Making my way to the kitchen for ice water or showering in the middle of the night just to cool down, was becoming a very strange nightly norm. The other awkward new norm was my incredible mood swings. I would try and hold my tongue when people pissed me off. I tried so hard to be graceful in conversations and then I would wake up to the internal silencing which I voiced as a scream, "Fuck this shit!", surprising myself and others in the process. This swing of emotions was both liberating and unnerving in equal measure.

There were times I couldn't catch my own breath. There was this dragon within me and she wanted to be birthed, was being birthed and once she was born, she invited all her families and friends to come on this ride with us.

Each of my mood swings, my manic moments, cascading memories represented a new dragon breathing so many different fires, but not just the devastating fires, but the incredibly powerful alchemising fires of feminine power which had been simmering and growing with each of my monthly cycles. These fires came, they fuelled my passions, my loves, my business, my voice and my entire world. And oftentimes it excited me on every level of my being. I was not going to be stopped,

I was not going to pause the power for a moment. And then the flames would be reduced to a flicker waiting for the next round of personal rocket fuel.

I knew this was a hormone adventure which was going to be a part of my life for the near future, at least for the next couple of years, and I could feel the realness of it.

Those rivers of the Amazon running down the side of my face, dripping down from my chin onto my clavicle and continuing their journey over the curve of my breasts into my cleavage and hitting my black lacy bra. When on other days the river Rhein flowed down from the nape of my neck, down between my shoulder blades, and down the curve my spine, tickling and making me roll my shoulders and sway my curvaceous hips – sometimes with a naughty smile to myself in remembrance as similar rivers of sweat.

And whilst in the heat of passionate moments the sweat making these journeys would be seen as sexy and highly desirable, the reality of a hot flash often feels anything but sexy and desirable!

This sweating was going to be a part of my life and I didn't care if it came whilst I was on stage speaking to audiences which included both men and women. It wouldn't care if I was with dignitaries or society members, or in the kitchen by myself making my sourdough bread. These sweats would visit me whilst I played with my grandchildren or sat making my way up piste on a ski lift. (Actually, being in the surroundings of a cold snowy mountain in the freezing cold seems to have been the biggest blessing in the years where my personal summers were running exceptionally hot!).

It's quite an experience to know that you are a living breathing moving oven that at any given moment you can explode into what feels like the blistering heat of 150°F. There's no need for an electric blanket, a rich thick duvet or even the highest thread count of the most luxurious cotton sheets. You are the heating system that keeps the bed, the room and the water in your home hot.

At the height of my menopause, I was in relationship with a kind man, a gentle soul who elegantly tried to make me aware of the intensity of my natural oven, not that I needed it, but the graciousness he offered made me grateful for his desire to be intimate with me in this way in these hot, sweaty and uncomfortable moments. Sometimes he would lie beside me in bed raising his hand and hovering it three feet above my belly and say, "You're having one now, aren't you?!?"

"YES! I was having "ONE"!!" screamed in my head and escaped in laughter with him.

Looking back now I wonder how intriguing and fascinating this must have been for him, and how it must be for men. Does it merit the same level of fascination for them as when they see our belly grow in pregnancy? Or does it intrigue them much as when they feel a baby move inside of us? What goes through a man's mind when he sees me transform, as I radiate in multiple ways during these special times in my life?

These furnace moments, which are commonly known as hot flashes, received many different names in my world. I started to turn it into an etymological adventure to find new ways of expressing the energy my body was exuding. "I'm having my own personal summer" had become one of my favourites.

"You can fry an egg on my belly" was another good one, which was only to be used in a very intimate setting. I started to realise that making fun of myself, making friends with the amazon rivers flowing from my body would become second nature to me. Embracing rather than being embarrassed by these moments and treating them as daily self-honouring rituals was the best way to dance through this dilemma. And trust me, it worked.

There were moments of frustration, emotional meltdowns, confusion, which led to even more resistance. Everything culminated in these massive surges in which the tapestry of my powerful situation was reminding me on a moment-by-moment basis the blessings of eldering.

Stepping out of these moments I knew the lack of education, or shall I say the lack of awareness, was a big part of my frustration.

Every time something happened in my body I was re-reminded of the fact that so many of us have no idea what's about to happen, and I mean that sincerely. Nor do we know, as mature women, when we're about to step into menopause. It just happens. My experience has been that we are not made aware by others, or our own bodies. There is no calendar, no road map, or timeline which we can consult in order to get ourselves physically, mentally and emotionally ready.

These hot flashes and rivers of sweat flowed with memories which would show up in my body, on my skin, on a deep cellular level, moments of growing up, of expectations, of confusion, of being unclean. Meanwhile, there was also a reminder of the lack of desire and passion which became a huge dragon that showed up every time to leave me in a state of despair.

Was this the end of my sensual life? Throughout my younger years I had developed a delicacy for sensual intimacy, was this also supposed to be over now?

A future without desire wasn't a future I wanted. It wasn't something "I was allowed" to speak freely about. I wanted this, this thing to be the thing I screamed to the sky and heavens above with the voice of an all-powerful woman.

As the rivers of sweat ensued It was like dramatic comedy, publicly pointing to this very present and wet occurrence in my life. Having my hormonal journey on full display for the world to see was a first for me. I had to wrap my head around this new reality. I found myself having a conversation with myself: "Liana, this is what's here. You're always mentoring others to BE with life exactly the way it is and exactly the way it isn't, so here you are, let's see if you can really walk your own talk!"

This part of the journey was as humbling as it was reassuring, all at the same time. I knew I could walk my own talk. With each step reclaimed a deeper level of empathy for myself as well as for other women who were discovering this fire. We were all discovering our own version of the fire breathing dragons, reacquainting ourselves with THAT powerful woman in the mirror on the wall, as well as our inner goddess.

What kept occurring for me here in these moments, was the recognition of a lack of learning for myself, and for others. Could or would it have been easier if I had had some guidance? Would I have been able to navigate these natural female tsunamis with more grace and acceptance? Could I have managed my moods with less drama, more magic, or simple surrender? How would we even know? How could we measure the difference when we don't even know ourselves? We won't know, not unless we start to share our experiences with one another, openly shamelessly… most of all proudly.

I'm not sure if today, my answer to this question would be totally truthful. We all know better after the fact. What I do know is that having experienced it the way I did, I am able to build a certain grid. This clear map if you will, which in co-creation with other unique maps, will show some of the way. YOU who have been through 'IT', can create a clearer possible understanding of the extraordinary dense desert of information to make the landscape fertile for generations of women, and men, to come.

It was within the art of all my alchemising fires that the devastation of self-containment, the liberation of the wise and wild woman within me came out to play. She brought with her a dance of many partners, one that had me second guessing myself in the mundane aspects of life as well as the woman I saw in the mirror. Some days I didn't recognise myself while looking at my reflection on the wall, or through my internal mirror. Some days it was foggy, with the recognition of self, gone. Other days the looking glass reflected back at me a woman radiating in her glorious power. Always reminding me to love myself even more than ever before, reminding me that I, Liana, my authentic essence was still there deep within, evolving into an even greater masterpiece than I could ever possibly imagine.

Without my tribe of women to guide me, to let me know what to expect, the deafening silence of women would continue. I … we wonderful women, would be forever in the dark about the gift these dragons of fire are blessing us with

And yet, on the days when the fog cleared, I knew I was being shown how to turn up the volume on my own soul. I was being invited to amplify my woman's voice so other women didn't have to experience the deafening silence. I was being given the gift of burning the old versions of myself, weaving together everything I had learned over the years, so this divine Centurion Woman, the one which kept appearing would remain with me. She would be the one to lead me through my rebirthing into the woman I am today.

The empowerment – which came from being brave so I could let go of the filters – came to me quietly. The empowerment of acknowledging that I am a divine being, just like YOU, that we as women are magnificent masterpieces blessed with this power to create life within us is beyond magical. We have access to this at every stage of our life – even if our wombs are no longer fertile, we are growing stronger with every conversation, in every private whisper with friends or on world stages we light up with our souls across the world.

As the filters were let go, and as the hot flashes subsided, there were moments I wondered if it was all over, if this part of my cycle was over. And then dragons of a different kind would announce themselves. The dragons of timidity, of anxiety and inner conflict. The dragons which made me question my worth, my passion for wonder, my whole reason for being.

These moments of being timid, nervous, wondering what or how to speak my silence, or asking for what I wanted, took me by surprise. "Liana is too timid" is not something anyone would ever say about me, but I recognised in the context of being me (boisterous, transparent and truthful) I could be the exact opposite within a split second. The thoughts raging through my mind mirrored the hormones which raged through my body, leaving me in a space of wanting to give all of my thoughts air, but I wouldn't say them out loud.

It was happening in my family life, in my business life and my romantic life. I felt I couldn't be too bold, too big, too loud, or too much woman; ultimately, I couldn't be 'too Liana'. It just wasn't ok. Too inappropriate, or too authentic – being too much of anything started to fall away. I found I'd had enough of silencing myself and once again I found myself just saying "Fuck it!" – but this time was different. This time was when I found myself becoming a guardian of grace, greatness and gratitude.

Learning to look at myself through the new lens of self, I came to trust my "determination transformations" which came through the alchemy of all my cultures. This helped me uncover, discover and recover my beautiful masterpiece called Liana Chaouli.

With oceans of emotions raging out loud while burning up the thoughts of being dirty, I started realising just how powerful we have always been and will be. I now understood that for the system of patriarchy, we women have always been too powerful, hence the silencing, the shaming of our bodies, our voices and our deepest desires. Our desires are a powerful engine to getting shit done! Suffocate a woman's desire and you shall silence her future.

The river of life may have stopped running through me, through us as we cycle through to the next phase of womanhood, but I soon realised through meditation that it never stops. It just changes, just like the rivers which never stop flowing until they reach the wide-open oceans. With this new sense of forever flowing, I asked myself why would I allow myself to be stopped, held back or even silenced? Why put my life, my career and my loves on hold, on pause whilst I navigated the rapids of this fast raging river?

Why should women be told when our rivers are to stop flowing? No one has the right to tell us when we must be silent! Why should we wise women of the world not show our wildness? Why should we as women not share our journeys, mapping them out for other women, so they too can navigate their way through the wilderness of twists and turns of this life unfolding?

Why should I hide the sweat pouring off my face while speaking to audiences from stages as I share my wisdom with those who have graciously come to listen to me? I believe that Authenticity IS our highest currency, we all have it, we can share if we so choose… yet why are we not circulating it freely into the world.

Why should I not share how I have gotten to this point of navigating the foggy and explosive journey of menopause with others? It is this generous authenticity which will pave the way for others to get bigger and show up in more transparent ways as well.

I am now one of the voices I longed to hear when I was a young girl. And whilst I may only be a few steps ahead of my sisters around the world, I choose to take my place on another stage – the one which gives me the chance to become the mentor, a part of the faculty in the Women's University which is so missing in the world.

Becoming Centurion and standing for all the things that I believed in, was and is a privilege. The invitation to rise up to tallness is so powerful. Without it standing in our strength, I realised, we become a cost to ourselves and others.

People are going to have an opinion about us anyway, and many will not like the fact that we embrace our fire. They are not going to want us to stand in our fire, our powerfulness. Yet I have realised that the more we shut down, the more they try to extinguish our fire, the more potent 'IT' becomes…. we become.

Coming to a place of understanding that the more we lean in, the more we warm hearts and souls, the more we return to self, keep the warmth inside of us, the more we create a power from which to grow and empower others. We GET TO share our stories, as we are here in this book for women – and men – for the world over to read – and we become the sovereign beings, the sovereign women building this much needed university, the faculties, the fountains of knowledge so many of us so desperately wanted yet didn't know where to find.

We need to change the narratives from ones of being dirty, shameful and silent to the ones who bring clarity and empowerment, because we are the one Sempais (the ones who have gone before). We shouldn't feel shameful about our bodies, the magic of how they work, nor should we be filled with guilt, or embarrassment by who we BE. We shouldn't be afraid of our ruby red flow. Nor should we fear the power which surges through us in our moments of wondering what the hell is going on within us, or around us.

Our value is within us. WE come fully equipped with everything we need in every stage of our lives. EVERYTHING we will ever need resides within us. We don't need to be filled up by someone else's greatness. We don't need other peoples' opinions of us to fulfil our vessel.

We have to learn to trust and believe that things are exactly how they are and how they are not. That this context of the validation and recognition from others requires us to play a role, a role which we can change in any given moment, choosing which parts of our life we want to take with us as we continue to weave this tapestry of life into the winter of our lives.

Our journey as a woman may have been passed down to us in negative messages due to the narrative of men: the men who fathered us, the men who were our doctors, our faith leaders, and our lovers, but we can change that. We can put their narrative on pause, take a breath and change it, but we must never stop our potent power in 'IT' tracks.

The negative narratives of 'menopausal women', the jokes of the "hormonal woman on the war path", the 'boss bitch' has to stop. Along with the belief we will one day be replaced for 'a younger model' because we were no longer worthy of desire, difficult to love, and far too sensitive to even have a conversation with to uncover what was really going on. We are worthy of desire; we are sensitive and we are difficult to love – and just like the birthing of a child is difficult, the love which follows is so deeply profound and nourishing, so richly rewarding.

We have to remember the men who try to love us, want to love us and who once desired us have also been given the harmful narrative we have been fed all our lives. This narrative runs so deep, deeper in societies and faiths, organisations and communities, that until we change the narrative, the damage will continually be done to families, and to humanity as a whole.

We were fed false truths about our bodies and how they worked to keep us in our place, to keep us small, to keep us from meddling in the world of men. And we are waking up to these falsehoods, remembering and sharing the real truths about ourselves.

The truths which are a part of the path and the reality of a BEING woman, any and all women. Like the fact that we have a vagina, breasts and are built to give birth. Like it is understood that we will have IT at some point in the autumn decades of our life, and that is all, all very matter of fact.

'IT' is to be accepted like the tides in the ocean and full moon nights which shower the world with magical source energy. Both hypnotic in their nature, and both deserving of moments where we take time to glance up or down in gratitude for these powerful energies we have been gifted.

'IT', I now understand, is a lot like the blessing of magical moon energy. 'IT' is a gift of transition, elevation, the path from frustration to freedom, a deep knowing, a rite of passage where we get to rise to the space of an Empress. All of us start as young princesses, grow into Goddesses as we dance through life and, somehow the most precious part of our powerful living journey is packed in societies screaming the silence of this Wisdom Gift.

We never got to read about this magical energy, this potent power of ours in books, nor did our girlfriends talk about it…none of that. But now we have this book, other books, opportunities like never before to make a difference in the lives of everyone on the planet.

Now in my sensual sixties, I smile to myself because I didn't ever think that I would write something about menopause and go way back to 1969 when I first got my period, but actually no pun intended…we have to go way, way, way back for all for us to really understand and listen to everything that is not being said about menopause, as well as what is being said.

This is our time to be the guides, the Centurions, the aunties, the voices and the reflection of power women are seeking deep within themselves. There is no time to stop and pause for a moment, because time waits for no woman. Time makes its own time and comes when IT wants to come.

All we have to do is show ourselves, share and support other women in the ways we needed, the ways they need and in ways which puts a new narrative of menopause on the treasure map of life.

Reflections

Reflections

Reflections

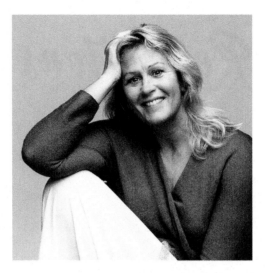

ULLIS KARLSSON
SWEDEN

After a severe burnout and being suicidal, Ulrika today shares her embodied wisdom with others.

With more than twenty-eight years of experience in traditional Western and Eastern Holistic disciplines – her expertise lies within Holistic Health, Personal Development, and Inner Leadership.

Ulrika's work as a Spiritual Teacher, Soul Coach, International Author, Yoga teacher/therapist takes her around the globe to work with women of different ages, from all levels of society.

Her vision is to contribute to a more balanced, harmonious, juicier, conscious, and loving world.

To find out more about Ullis and the work she does, and how to work with her visit https://ulliskarlsson.com

Chapter Eleven

HAPPY, HORNY, AND IN HARMONY: MAGICAL MOMENTS OF MENOPAUSE

Congratulations to you to have this book in your hands. The frequency and the energy of this book has attracted You, and Your energy has consciously – or unconsciously – attracted her into your energetic field. It is truly something special to read a book designed for women – created by women with different frequencies and energetic signatures. This book is a tasty buffet with different dishes, exotic colours, and flavours. Take what resonates with you – what you crave for the moment – and let the other dishes and flavours be for another time.

WHO AM I WHO SHARES MY ENERGY – AND MY STORY – WITH YOU IN THIS CHAPTER?

My name is Ulrika Karlsson, I am born and raised in beautiful Sweden. The home of the Vikings, and the beautiful Aurora Borealis – just to mention some well-known things from the energetic imprints surrounding me. I write this chapter in early 2022. It is winter here in Sweden, it is pitch black and cold outside. The outer world – as we have known it – is on fire, and upside down since spring 2020.

The Swedish energetic imprints can be perceived as polarities in menopause – both the fierce and fiery energy of the Vikings, and the beautiful flow of Northern Lights of Aurora Borealis. Masculine and Feminine. Fire and Water. Menopause does not have to be all fires – like hot flushes – it can be beautiful and flowing as Aurora Borealis, and everything between.

The combination of experiencing menopause as a single mum with two teenagers has been quite an emotional rollercoaster. Luckily, Yoga, being out in nature and hanging out with my beloved ones have been my Lifesavers during this important initiation and transformation into the "Crown energy" (described later).

I have a very special relation with the water element – as one aspect of me is a mermaid. In my book 'Holy F*ck and Sacred Water', I share more about it. As we all contain of mainly water, menopause is a time that affects the quality of our inner waters. The balance between the water and fire element therefore influences our ability to be happy, horny, and harmonious.

As a Yogi, balance and harmony is the key to be happy. When we, as women are happy and relaxed it is easier to be horny. So, let's explore a bit of the yogic perspectives on menopause.

ENERGIES AND CHAKRAS – FROM THE YOGIC PERSPECTIVE

My perception is that *everything* is energy, and we are all "Spiritual Beings, in physical energetical bodies, containing all elements – Earth, Water, Fire, Air, Ether.

Everything we experience is energy vibrating at different frequencies. Our bodies are energy – made of energy – and the world we perceive and experience we live in, is energy. So, some of these things I write about here – are from an energetic yogic perspective. Yoga literally just means "union", a unification and connection of all energies of self and others.

Energy moves through the body through energetic so-called Meridians. In the Yogic aspect, our physical human bodies contain of chakras – or energy centres. Each chakra represents different kinds of energies, with different elements and polarities, and each one is connected to the central nervous system and the endocrine hormone system. They are also associated with a specific sense, hormonal gland, a specific body part, colour, energies, and polarities etc.

The three lower chakras – the root chakra, the sexual chakra and the solar plexus chakra – represents our subconscious, or unconscious mind. The heart, throat, third eye and crown chakra represents our conscious mind. They are unconsciously governed by the three lower chakras. They are all connected to and communicate with each other.

So, for me, as energetical beings, our energy "needs a place to hang out and play, and to experience this 3D reality". That is why we have been given these amazing "physical" and complexed designed bodies. Energetically speaking our bodies are in a denser reality – "Matrix", which is the third dimensional field. Our souls are in the fifth dimensional field and above. The experience we have as souls, within our physical bodies and the lives we live here as we "walk in our shoes" – there are a lot of polarities in the third dimension to experience. "Good-bad, Love-fear, Pain-Pleasure, Ease-Disease, Men-Women" etc. This is what we call "Life" here on Earth.

However, while we live here on mother earth, our *physical bodies are the vessel* where our Divine Soul resides. For our amazing bodies to be in harmony, there are many complex systems that work together as a whole. *Each cell, body part, organ, chakra, complex system in itself – such as the nervous system and the endocrine hormone system – plays a significant role in our quality of Life. During menopause these systems are supposed to transition us into a more relaxed state of being. However, due to all inner and external stress factors most of us experience – menopause is anything but smooth and relaxing. Everything in the body has it own's unique assignment, as they all connect, rely and depend on each other. The human body is indeed a complex, beautiful and magical design – it is our temple – created by Divine Source.*

For us women cycles and phases are a natural part of our lives – as we follow the natural phases of the moon. Our hormone system – connected to and with help from the nervous system – regulates and control these phases of Life. For instance, when it is time to give birth, transition from a girl into womanhood – and from a fertile woman into the magical menopause.

In our everyday life most of us take for granted that we can automatically function "normally". All these systems are managed unconsciously – working together – in union. For instance, the hormone system regulates automatically – when it is time to go to sleep – or when we are hungry. It also creates the "juiciness" we feel when we are horny, or not – or sexually satisfied, or not. Hormones regulates menstruation – or Moon Blood – for us women. During menopause, these systems – just like the computer is upgraded to a newer version – our energetical systems are upgraded too. As we chaotically upgrade, we energetically evolve – from chaos comes magical order. In the midst of chaos of my menopause – knowing this became a lifeline to relax into.

From my yogic perception, we are energy that never dies – it just takes different shapes, forms, and transforms as we move through life. *However, when it comes to energy – regardless of what form of energy it is – for energy to flow naturally and limitlessly, it needs to be balanced. How we give and how we receive – balanced in Feminine and Masculine – as a whole. We receive and transmit energy at the same time – all the time.*

In the yogic perspective, when we as women are in our fertile phase, we "leak our energy" every month as we leak blood. It is like a "small death" – where we as women really should just rest more. Be more contemplative and move our focus inwards. *To just Be more – yet we often end up to Do more.* Instead, we who are mothers focus on our babies and children as they are growing up. As a mother, I realised that I lost myself as I nurtured and nourished my children – and focused on their needs and wants – more than I tended to my own. I did it freely by choice, from love – yet it was still a leakage of my energy. I gave more love, time, attention, energy etc. – than I could receive. This imbalance between giving and receiving created stress, it made me depressed and "dry as a desert". *Many of us unconsciously forget to fill up our own cup – before we give it to others. This basically means we leak quite a lot of energy on an everyday base – over time.* Chronic stress is known to activate and trigger menopause early – and create more/severe symptoms.

It is at times like these when, complex designed systems, are out of balance, in dis-ease – or in different readjustment phases – our bodies make sure we pay attention to them. It is an opportunity for us to reconnect us back into ourselves. That the natural cycles of life – or unexpected and unpredicted things and events – "just happens to us". Or maybe happens for us? As I entered menopause, my body did not work and function as I was used to – or as I wanted it to. I did not recognise my body as I gained weight no matter what I ate or how much I exercised. I did not recognise my emotions and behaviours, as I experienced an emotional roller coaster every day. I could go from happy to unhappy – harmonious to un-ease. From one day to another, I found myself in totally new experiences – and they influenced and changed my whole Life – or rather my perception of life. And I found myself in totally new and unknown territory.

OUTER TRIGGERS FOR INNER CHANGES

In the yogic perspective this period – since spring 2020 – is a massive awakening. It is manifesting in a physical form as we need to experience everything that comes with it. As we experience all the fears etc, we can transform it and thereby raise our frequency. It is quite mind blowing that I never in my lifetime heard about so many women activated menopause at the same time as now, myself included. What we experience during this intense and challenging period is simply here to aid humankind evolve into a higher state of consciousness – it is a gift in disguise. We need to wake up from our individual and collective slumber – and take radical responsibility for how we treat ourselves, others, and this beautiful planet that we call home. Chaotic times are – just like menopause – part of the natural evolution of our souls. It is safe to say that we all have experienced different outer – and inner – challenges during this period.

As a Yogi, I have known for a very long time that this ascension time would come. That everything familiar first should crumble and fall – and then fall into place. This is going to be the end for old outdated systems and the beginning of something new – to co create something better. Just like menopause transitions us into a higher version of ourselves. We need to let the older versions to die – to be reborn wiser, happier and more balanced. We will never go back to "normal", as "normal" was not beneficiary for everybody – and nor was it sustainable for our planet. I just did not know in what shape this shift in consciousness – would look like. I really felt it coming though – in every cell of my body – long before it played itself out.

For me personally this has been a very challenging time in so many ways. I lost my business, as in my Yoga studio – my economical lifeline – right before this whole thing started spring 2020. As a single mum of two teenagers, I have responsibilities for them as well. It was very scary and triggered a lot of old unconscious fears and wounds within me. I was never afraid of what was going on in itself – but I felt the collective fears and the heaviness in energy. Being an introvert empath I felt the collective fears so intense in my own physical body that it felt like a deep depression. The experience was very heavy and intense. To me it felt like an apocalypse was here. The outer chaos – and economical worries for my family – triggered my weak and vulnerable spot, my sleep. I started to lose sleep and I found myself once again lying awake most nights with a stressed mind (Read more in my autobiography *2:47 am The Journey Home to My Heart*).

"I get out of bed and walk into the bathroom, where I find myself in front of the bathroom mirror. I can barely look into my own eyes as I am filled with so much self-contempt. It's quiet and everyone except me is asleep. I move in a quiet and familiar way in the dark. I walk into my beloved children's bedroom and lie next to them, one at a time for a while. Feeling their warm little bodies. Crawling close, very close. Trying to get some of the warmth and calm they radiate. I know I will not be able to fall asleep again" – excerpt from "*2:47 am The Journey Home to My Heart*".

These sleepless nights quite quickly took its toll on me, I felt stressed, worried, and unhappy during the day. I also noticed different symptoms in my body. I felt an inner heaviness and sort of a depression. Like a "small death". My *Moon Blood* started to be irregular, and one month it did not come at all – and it never came back. It was like a loss of a long-time friend where I did not have a chance to say a proper goodbye to. I did not get a chance to do a proper ceremony, or something, to thank and honour the beautiful function and flow of my body that it had provided for me over my Life. *My Moon Blood* that had been me for more than thirty-five years – with its ability to tell me when I was ready to become pregnant had ended. Such a truly amazing gift as a woman – the experience to become pregnant – and create new Life was now gone. So, I grieved over the sudden loss of my *Moon Blood* for a while. The culmination of these stress factors triggered me into – what I after a while realised – my menopause.

From here, there were many changes, and a lot of different things happened more or less simultaneously. I gained four kilos in four weeks. These extra kilos decorated itself – without my consent – as a "fluff" over my ovaries and the lower part of my belly. I felt bloated and sore. There was a constant yet dull pain in my ovaries – and my breasts felt heavy and very tender. Suddenly just like that, I got hot flashes at nights. They came in "waves" three – four times per night and they made me so hot and sweaty. And those hot waves made it even more impossible to sleep, as I laid there in my cold and damp sheets. If I was emotional and sensitive before my menopause – my emotions took me on a rollercoaster and enhanced the experience and the emotions tenfold. One day could be like a full year in different seasons. I laughed, and I cried unexpectedly just like that. I got angry, excited, and then very tired and exhausted, also out of the blue. I experienced brain fog. Every day was like an adventure. I never knew what was coming and I did not recognise myself – or the processes going on inside of my body. I mean, even if I obviously always had known that this day was going to come, it happened almost from one day to another. I was simply not prepared for this big Life change. On top of this, I completely lost "appetite" for sex and my libido. I had no feeling of "juiciness" at all. This lack of "juice" made me feel unhappy, out of balance and tense. There was no magic left.

HORMONE YOGA, YIN AND YANG ENERGIES

However, I was in a very fortunate position with so many different tools! Over my twenty-eight years when I have studied and explored various holistic disciplines and different Yoga forms – I have designed and developed *Yoga for empaths and Hormone Yoga for lust and sensuality. In Hormone Yoga we can increase our inner flow and libido. It is designed to balance our intricate and delicate female hormones– regardless of what phase in life we are in – as the wonderful women we are.*

With a background as a Yoga teacher in many yogic disciplines – Ashtanga Vinyasa, Hatha Yoga, Yin Yoga, Yoga Therapy etc. Hormone Yoga is truly something extra ordinary. It is a combination of so many different healing modalities. It also developed through my own long quest and experience from healing myself from my long-time depression and burn out (read more in *2:47 am The Journey Home to My Heart*). At the time when I was depressed there were mainly Yoga disciplines with very much energy of the masculine essence – Yang energy – on the market. They were too hard for my body, mind and spirit at the time. They made me even more depleted and depressed. So, over some time Yoga for empaths, and the Hormone Yoga "came intuitively through me" – through my own needs to recover from stress, burn out, depression and depletion.

In Hormone Yoga we connect to the glands, conscious breaths, sounds and mantras etc. – this intuitive Yoga is in tuned with the subtle – yet very potent feminine essence of Yin.

We all have both yin and yang energy within us, regardless of gender. *Yin is the feminine energy where Yang is the masculine energy.* These two polarities need each other to function in balance, harmony and communication – to work as a whole "unity". The polarities of yin and yang co-relate, co-create and communicate with each other – as they create movement. Movement in the physical, mental and emotional body – and movement of Life itself. Everything in Universe is created by these different polarities – like expansion and contraction, Sun and Moon, and Masculine and Feminine etc.

Basically, and generally speaking – we as women in female physical bodies have a bit more of the yin essence. And, generally – men in male bodies have more of the yang energy.

Over centuries an unconscious imbalance has been created between the feminine and the masculine energies. A lot of what is associated with the Divine Feminine has been suppressed and distorted. A lot of what is associated with the Divine Masculine have also been distorted yet enhanced. This unconscious imbalance has created a disconnection from Divinity. Disconnection and distortion from; the Sacred Union of the Feminine and Masculine, within ourselves, each other, and Mother Earth.

When separated and disconnected we never feel that we are whole. To be whole, happy, horny, and harmonious, requires a reconnection of the good, bad, the shadows and the light.

WESTERN SOCIETIES AND ENERGIES HERE

In our Western societies, these unconscious disconnections, are more visible and tangible than in many Eastern societies – as Eastern societies have a more holistic approach on Body-Mind-Spirit.

In the Western and Northern hemisphere, we have a lot of focus on *Doing. And it is a lot about doing in the external realm, which pretty much is associated with the essence of the masculine energy.* We focus on materialistic things, our superficial appearance and look. A lot of energy is spent on how we want to be perceived by others. Many women spend a lot of energy and time and might feel an urge to "make themselves up" – with a lot of makeup. As I entered menopause, my old habits and eating disorders were triggered as my appearance and look changed. This gave me a new opportunity to look deeper once again – into old wounds and shadows – and transform them into magical gifts.

We also tend to have a lot of focus on our careers – and/or on the importance to have a "higher education". We want to climb the career ladder, to move up in higher positions. We focus a lot on money. How we can have more, earn more. *How we can buy more and do more.* We want to have more and greater experiences, more travels – more of everything. We strive to be more productive, efficient, and successful. We focus very much on the external world. We seek outer acknowledgement. We fill our body-mind-spirit every day in and every day out with different outer stimuli and distractions. We fill our already busy calendars, busy minds, and lives, with even more activities – as we believe the "more the better". What we don't realise is that all this focus on the external appearances and realms creates more stress, disconnection, and disharmony. Again, the more unconscious stress we have stored in our bodies – the more uncomfortable symptoms we experience during menopause. For me, the stress that came with lack of career and inflow of money – certainly affected my menopausal symptoms for the worse.

Many of us try so hard – we push ourselves – to fit into what is "considered to be normal". I know for sure that I have done that my whole Life – and this behaviour have affected my health, thought processes, balance and happiness levels. What is normal? And who gets to decide what is normal? "Normal" is a norm – a designed thought form of what we should or should not do – that a few people decided on how to be "normal" and ordinary. Who wants to be ordinary anyway?

We try our best just to be normal and included – as we just want to belong. We do as we are told, stand in lines and we don't rock the boat. In our modern societies – everything moves faster and faster with more outer impressions, "shoulds" and distractions – we are increasingly stressed and disconnected. The unnatural tempo we have created for ourselves leave us, in state of being where most of us are not balanced, present – or happy. We unconsciously take ourselves from the present moment and we move into the future – the next activity, thought, "quick fix", distraction, or instant gratification – the next thing we can do. The more Doing – the less Being. The less we are Being in the present moment – the less access we have to be happy, horny and in harmony. *It is in the moment that magic happens.* In menopause we are given the opportunity to relax more into ourselves, with less obligations and responsibility for others. Here, Yoga is an essential tool for me to balance the fire of doing and the flow of being.

We are constantly doing things, either physically or mentally as we want to solve another problem – and we want to be in control. We would like to believe that we are on top of things, when we are, in fact not. Being "in control" is merely an illusion created by us. When the symptoms of my menopause peaked, I literally had no control over my emotional rollercoaster – or my mood swings. I was in the illusion that my depression and everything I had been through in my life had given me the lessons needed so I would not have to go through big emotional swings again. That the balance I had created in my life – somehow was going to be status quo.

The thing is, when we are in constant motion and doing things – physically or mentally – we move the energy upwards in an ascending flow. This is the masculine energy where we tend to disconnect from our bodies and become more "mental" and logical. All in the strive to be more successful – we over-think *"how to do it"*. We then unconsciously move the energy out from our Hearts into our headspace. Over the centuries, this has become an imbalance in energetic flow – and a dysfunctional aspect – in our part of the world. We simply live to much in our "headspace" and are disconnected from our bodies – and with that our "juiciness" and libidos. *However, as we move in the ascending flow we evolve into the energy of crown chakra – where we have access to all the chakras and their storage of challenges and gifts. Many women in menopause, myself included, experience new opportunities to embrace our new bodies. The more we embrace ourselves – the more access we have to be horny, happy and in harmony.*

We do know stress day in, and day out affects us negatively. As we live too much in the "unconscious" masculine energy – without balance to the feminine, this affects us on all levels; physical, emotional, mental, spiritual – and sexual. Not only does our modern lifestyle disempower and disconnect us – it also makes us unhappy, unbalanced and leave us with dis-ease. We seem to have lost the deep connection to Mother Earth as well – and we don't follow and honour the natural, organic cycles – and flow of nature. All seasons influence our nervous system, our hormone system, our chakra system, our inner organs etc. – our whole body-mind-spirit – as energetic beings.

Take the month of December and Christian celebration of Christmas as a perfect example. Here in Sweden this is the darkest month of the entire year. We only have an average of six hours of daylight. If we would be in balance with nature and its natural organic flow – we would simply follow and do like nature does. To slow down. To sleep more – to move inwards, contemplate more.

Instead, many of us, run around more stressed than ever. Many businesses have their annual closing with stressful deadlines. I used to stress home to pick up my kids, clean, decorate, cook to prepare for the holidays. I was all fired up and stressed to buy the perfect Christmas gifts. I went to Christmas dinners and parties drinking and socialising – the total opposite what my body truly needed. I visited so many relatives, I was depleted and needed a week´s vacation after the holidays.

HOW DOES ALL THIS STRESS AFFECT US?

Our autonomous nervous system is originally designed to maintain a good balance in our inner environment. It consists of the *sympathetic and the parasympathetic nervous system*. The *sympathetic nervous system is like our defence system*, it is activated when we are in danger – or in a perceived danger – and when we need more energy to fight, or to flee. This releases a "cocktail" of stress hormones – cortisol, adrenalin, and noradrenaline – within us. *The Yang – Masculine – energy represents the sympathetic nervous system*. The *element* for Yang is *fire*.

When we are in conscious – or unconscious – stress we are automatically in the influence of the sympathetic nervous system. All our inner organs, our nervous system and hormone system is in automatic unconscious "fight or flight mode" – as we are "all fired up". The stress hormones pumps through our blood and influence all aspects of us – simply to produce more power. As we need more energy, more "fire", to take the necessary action of fight or flight.

The sympathetic nervous system is designed so we can use the accumulated energy – as generated power – for survival. This accumulated fire energy is stored within our bodies. As we live, quite unconsciously, stressful lifestyles our sympathetic nervous system is on fire – more or less – all the time. "We feed fire with fire". In our societies, we also compare and compete a lot. We create things to stress about, and the more stressed we are the more stress we attract. It is like a downward negative spiral – which is most peoples "natural yet very unnatural and unconscious state of being". Over an extended period of time, the repetition of stress, even if there is a low stress factor – causes a lot of stress related symptoms and dis-eases – not being at ease. For me, all this fire created a burnout, depression, and severe sleeping disorders. As I entered menopause, the fear of being burnt out and depressed reappeared.

With too much fire in the energy system, it creates inflammations in body-mind-spirit. We believe that this stressed state of being in "Matrix" is a proof that we are "busy being successful and good citizens". This whole conception is merely an illusion and is far from the truth of who we are – instead more stress is stored.

From an energetic perspective this is why many have stress related symptoms – depression, poor sleep, burn outs, IBS, cancer, poor libido, heart dis-eases etc. We are depleted and burned out from too much fire.

For us women in female bodies, with sensitive reproductive organs this unconscious stressful Yang energy is even more harmful. Our essence is more of the Feminine energy – *Yin* – which *is the descending flow.* The descending flow moves us into our sexual chakra – womb space – where we connect to our sexuality and to Mother Earth. *Yin represents the parasympathetic nervous system – where water is the element. Water includes all kind of bodily fluids – like spinal fluids, in the fascia (that surrounds eighty per cent of our muscle tissues), blood, urine, semen, female orgasms etc. There are many important connections between Yoni, Lingam and the Heart – the water element – as in blood is just one of them. Yoni for women – which is the Vagina – means "Divine Portal, or Sacred Passage". Lingam for men, means "Pillar of Light". Our genitals are part of our* sexual chakra *– highly associated with water – as in flow, moist, juiciness, being horny, and the ability to have fountain orgasms and ejaculations...*

The heart chakra is the centre where the ascending and descending flow of the Masculine and Feminine connects in a harmonious dance and Sacred union. It nourishes and nurture with compassion and unconditional Love. Therefore, it is so important, for men and women, to descend from the "mental headspace" – and flow into the Heart, and the womb space. Here we reconnect with ourselves.

When we are connected in the heart – instead of stress and fears – love pumps and flows into our veins. From love, we create a more balanced, happier, and harmonious world for all of us to live in together. *The heart is very much associated with the thymus gland, and with the element of air.* Air as in space – space to breath and to expand, as to create a space from where we can expand our love, to love ourselves and others. God knows this world needs much more love! I have realised that not loving myself was a big reason for my burn out. To flood myself with love and compassion is an excellent tool to flush out the excess fire to create balance. While entering menopause a tsunami of overwhelming emotions came over me. This gave me a new opportunity to love myself even more.

It is also important to be connected in heart while making love – as the blood pumps through the heart into yoni and lingam. If not connected in our hearts – as when we are too stressed and disconnected – it creates unconscious traumas and imbalances for both men and women (read more in my book *Holy F*ck and Sacred Water*). This indicates the necessity for us women to be relaxed to enjoy sex, while men generally can use sex as a stress release.

The parasympathetic nervous system is what clears out toxics and "flushes out" waste, it cleanses, and it soothes. It is the part of the nervous system that rebuilds our cells, our bodies and to counteract the effects of the sympathetic nervous system. It is essential that the nervous system, as well as the hormonal system is in balance for our wellbeing, for our health. It is also responsible for stimulation of "rest-and-digest" or "feed and breed" activities that occur when the body is at rest, especially after eating, including sexual arousal, salivation, lubrication (mucous membranes in yoni), lacrimation (as in tears), urination, digestion, and defecation. No water – no "juiciness".

The more we are doing – the less we are being. The more stress – the less "juice".

Most of us don't fully relax into the parasympathetic nervous system for as long, or as deep as we would need to be. *We don't access oxytocin ("the love and bonding hormone"), serotonin ("mood and sleep hormone"), dopamine ("feel good hormone") and endorphins ("pain relief hormone") when in constant stress. As we are all fired up by constantly doing one activity or another. Mentally or physically.*

Stress influences the adrenals – which become burned out and depleted. Another medical term for burned out is, adrenal fatigue.

Adrenals are in the yogic perspective, connected to the root chakra – which is about survival and being grounded, or rooted in oneself. As in being connected within in body-mind-spirit, to others and to Mother Earth. When stressed, we are not grounded – nor connected – as the energy is more up in "the headspace" rather than in the body. The element of the root chakra is *soil. That is why it is so essential to ground ourselves in our busy societies – the more stressed we are the more we need to ground ourselves.*

Adrenals are also connected to the solar plexus chakra, which is associated to the Masculine Yang energy. It is also called "the fire chakra" and is associated with doing – as it is an extrovert chakra where we also connect with others. Because all this masculine fire, our inner organs and fascia, as well as the mucous membrane in Yoni dries up as the water leaves. Yoni's natural moist and juiciness "shrivel and shut down". We become dry, disconnected and we lose our inner flow and the "juiciness" of our libido. Due to our unbalanced lifestyles we women unconsciously store a lot of stress and tension in our ovaries, the uterus and yonis. This causes a disconnection to our hearts and yonis, our sexuality, lust and sex life. In menopause the stored stress is what causes a lot of its symptoms – as it all comes to the surface. When we release the stress and become more balanced the symptoms "flushes out". Menopause, when embraced create juicy magic.

MENOPAUSE FROM THE YOGIC PERSPECTIVE

Cycles and phases are such an important and natural part of what women experience – and always have been. Each cycle is beautiful and comes with Divine significance. Through centuries wise women shared their accumulated wisdom, insights, Moon Blood ceremonies and ancient medicine with their tribe – gathered around sacred bonfires. That was how the teachings and initiations was inherited and passed throughout the blood lineages. These sacred gatherings played such a vital role for women of all ages. It connected them to their own inner wisdom – as well as the wisdom of their ancestorial Spirits. In traditional Eastern societies the wise and the elder women are still consciously honoured and respected.

We should truly celebrate our natural and sacred cycles more here in the West, as they do in many other traditional civilisations. We have truly, and sadly unconsciously lost it all. Not only the sacred gatherings in itself – but all the connections, the perception upon Moon Blood, the inherited wisdom that came with them. When we enter menopause and the Moon Blood stops many of us experience rejection, shame – discarded as we are being too old. In Sweden there is even a negative word and energy for it – "Being a menopause cow". We tend to hide our natural phases, joke about them, or be ashamed of them. We also have a distorted view upon ageing – like it is a condition that "needs to be fixed or controlled". This perception truly disempowers and disconnect us, from our Feminine essence.

In yogic perspective, menopause comes with a magical transition – into energetic, emotional, mental, sexual and Spiritual shifts. Shifts that evolves us into our wise woman years and brings us into the majestic and magical crown chakra. It is all about being the embodied insights and wisdom, where we wear the crown of wisdom.

Through our lives, we experience distinct phases as we ascend in the chakra system – through the different chakras. Each chakra has its different Life themes – with its own unique energy and polarity. The changes in our chakras reflect many of the changes in our physical body. During menopause, we are often guided to reconnect to themes from earlier in our lives – things we have left unexplored – or wounds who have not healed. When we rise to the challenge, we come to own a new mature relationship to our body, our intuition, our sexuality, our spiritual selves, our sacredness – and wholeness. I had to face some old wounds – or illusions – such as my perception of my body and feelings of "not being beautiful and worthy enough".

One way to manage this challenge – is to reflect upon how the Life experiences you have during menopause corresponds to the different chakras and their themes. Reflect upon how they relate to your past, especially your childhood – what has been left unresolved?

Have you unconsciously buried fears as they are stored deep within your physical body in the different chakras?

Or alternatively, do you experience health problems related to any of the chakras?

As I entered menopause, I needed to let go of even more of my expectations on "how it should be" and practice more acceptance of myself. To be more heart cantered with love and compassion for myself – whilst trying to figure out how to keep balanced and in harmony with a "new" body and circumstances. I reflected a lot upon questions such as: *"Who am I when my teenagers don't need me anymore? What is my new role, my purpose? How can I accept my new body?"* And the realisation that all the love and energy I have given to my children, I can now focus it more into me. *"How shall I channel this extra energy into the world?*

The crown chakra is an entrance to universal energy and wisdom. It is a higher perspective. It is completion. It magical, majestical and comes with a deep inner knowing and intuition – that you are whole and connected with everything.

As our physical bodies mature and relax into the majestic and magical crown – our physical energetic vessel is more whole and contained. We are in completion – with no more unconscious need to compare or compete with anybody. There are no more energy leakages caused by Moon Blood. No more being over responsible for children. Not so many chores to attend to, not so many needs to tend to – but ourselves. *We fill our vessel up with ourselves and our needs, with more of what we like to do and less "must do's".* We get more access to our own energy, our power. More access to what makes us happy and harmonious. More time, and less stress can make us reconnect to what makes us horny, and how we want to be sexually satisfied. Magical moments after menopause awaits us ladies.

As we relax more into presence, more into our bodies – and into the **parasympathetic** nervous system – stored stress and tension transforms. *We see it as our muscles tend to be softer and we get more wrinkles – as the water element is released from previously stressed organs and tissues. The water element obviously moves more freely in bodies that are not tight from stress – meaning we have more access to our juiciness and our libido.*

The energetic and important transitions for a woman in this time of her life – can manifest in so many ways – depending on who we are and what we have stored. Hormone Yoga is one holistic discipline that can make this transition so much easier.

When energy flows more freely through our physical body we experience a deeper connection to spirit and spiritual gifts like intuition – which is a magical key part of the wise woman archetype. Our ability to sense and connect with energies and spirit is increased. This connection is something that can continue to deepen for the rest of our lives. *This is conscious ageing to me – to embrace the transition and focus on our inner wisdom, insights and juiciness gained. It is a new birth, a transition into our higher selves, and to fully own the crown's energy is a magical and majestic experience – if we embrace it as such. I love to explore and go even deeper into these aspects of myself.*

In other words, the crown chakra is an entrance to universal energy and wisdom. It is a higher perspective. It is completion. It is magical, majestical and comes with a deep inner knowing and intuition – that you are whole and connected with everything.

HAPPY, HORNY, AND IN HARMONY – MAGICAL MOMENTS DURING AND AFTER MENOPAUSE

So, as I was triggered by outer circumstances into the phase of my own crown, I started to do what I guide others through – I did my Hormone Yoga. I listened to my own pre-recorded Hormone Yoga classes. After only three weeks I noticed many improvements in body, mind and spirit. My body was less bloated, and less sore. My breasts were less heavy and tender – and the dull pain in my ovaries disappeared. My hot flushes "evaporated" just like that and vanished as quickly as they came. My emotions were more stable, and my sleep was improved. My weight adjusted itself more to my ideal weight. I felt more balanced, happier, more in harmony, with more juiciness – and my lust and libido were back.

Here I am now, on the other side of menopause. I am happy, horny, sexually satisfied and in harmony in body, mind and spirit. In hormonal balance – enjoying the magical moments after menopause. I am here – reconnected to my inner power, wisdom, juiciness and libido. In balance with the flow, and beauty of the Feminine. The Feminine associated with the dancing Northern lights of Aurora Borealis. with its green colours of the Heart chakra, and purple colours of the crown chakra. In balance with the fiery energy of the Masculine Vikings. In balance and harmony with all the elements inside and outside of me. This reminds me of my healing journey I share in the chapter Dark F*ck: "Holy F*ck and Sacred Water – The Secret Connections to Everything"

"My soft tears on my cheeks and the sacred water from my yoni were now flowing in harmony, in synchronicity. Now my water originated from pure gratitude, instead of pain, despair, rage, and fury. I felt such gratitude for this long-lost, unknown, and unconscious connection in a holy f*ck. I was grateful for being swept away by the amazing water. Grateful for my flow, and for allowing myself to flow through every aspect of life. Grateful to reclaim another aspect of myself, with the precious help from my sacred water. Grateful for feeling so much love toward myself. I felt such gratitude to my teacher for making this possible. I flowed in gratitude.

"*The sacred water, the same essence as the feminine and as spirit itself, moves in mysterious ways through the most solid forms of all kinds of resistance and obstacles. It transforms all our accumulated fears, all of our resistance, into a flowing river of freedom and abundance.*" – excerpt from "Holy F*ck and Sacred Water – The Secret Connections to Everything".

In the end, the real wisdom of menopause may be to come back home to yourself and find balance, harmony, your inner wisdom, and your sacred crown – and wear it as you own it.

If there is only one sentence, or even one word, in this chapter that resonates with you – it will ripple out to your inner environment and create a hormonal influence. When you are in hormonal balance your energy ripple out and influences others. This ripple effect is how we together can create a more balanced world where we all can thrive. *Where we all can be happy, horny, in harmony and enjoying the juicy and magical moments during and after menopause.*

Reflections

Reflections

About the Publisher

A UK based boutique publishing house which specialises in changing the mainstream narratives through the art of literature. Titles published incorporate solo authors as well as a carefully chosen groups of individuals for a wide variety of anthologies in the realms of human rights, social change and cultural diversity.

As well as being an international bestselling author, writer, authority coach, educator and publisher, founder of *Dawn Publishing* Dawn Bates, specialises in developing brand expansion strategies and global visions, underpinned with powerful leadership and profound truths.

She writes for various magazines, and when not travelling or sailing around the world on yachts, she appears on multiple media channels highlighting and discussing essential subjects in today's society.

All the titles published under the *Dawn Publishing* brand bring together the multi-faceted aspects of the world we live in and take you on a rollercoaster ride of emotions while delivering mic dropping inspiration, motivation, and awakening. The books capture life around the world in all its rawness.

Discover more books from *Dawn Publishing* by visiting: www.dawnbates.com/readers

Printed in Great Britain
by Amazon

80622234R00161